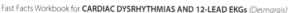

Fast Facts for the **NEONATAL NURSE**: Care Essentials for Normal and High-Risk Neonates, Second Edition *(Davidson)*

Fast Facts About **NEUROCRITICAL CARE**: A Quick Reference for the Advanced Practice Provider *(McLaughlin)*

Fast Facts for the **NEW NURSE PRACTITIONER**: What You Really Need to Know, Second Edition *(Aktan)*

Fast Facts for **NURSE PRACTITIONERS:** Practice Essentials for Clinical Subspecialties *(Aktan)*

Fast Facts for the **NURSE PRECEPTOR**: Keys to Providing a Successful Preceptorship, Second Edition *(Ciocco)*

Fast Facts for the **NURSE PSYCHOTHERAPIST**: The Process of Becoming *(Jones, Tusaie)*

Fast Facts About **NURSING AND THE LAW**: Law for Nurses *(Grant, Ballard)*

Fast Facts About the **NURSING PROFESSION**: Historical Perspectives *(Hunt)*

Fast Facts for the **OPERATING ROOM NURSE**: An Orientation and Care Guide, Second Edition *(Criscitelli)*

Fast Facts for the **PEDIATRIC NURSE**: An Orientation Guide *(Rupert, Young)*

Fast Facts Handbook for **PEDIATRIC PRIMARY CARE:** A Guide for Nurse Practitioners and Physician Assistants *(Ruggiero, Ruggiero)*

Fast Facts About **PRESSURE ULCER CARE FOR NURSES**: How to Prevent, Detect, and Resolve Them *(Dziedzic)*

Fast Facts About **PTSD**: A Guide for Nurses and Other Health Care Professionals *(Adams)*

Fast Facts for the **RADIOLOGY NURSE**: An Orientation and Nursing Care Guide, Second Edition *(Grossman)*

Fast Facts About **RELIGION FOR NURSES**: Implications for Patient Care *(Taylor)*

Fast Facts for the **SCHOOL NURSE**: What You Need to Know, Third Edition *(Loschiavo)*

Fast Facts About **SEXUALLY TRANSMITTED INFECTIONS**: A Nurse's Guide to Expert Patient Care *(Scannell)*

Fast Facts for **STROKE CARE NURSING**: An Expert Care Guide, Second Edition *(Morrison)*

Fast Facts for the **STUDENT NURSE**: Nursing Student Success *(Stabler-Haas)*

Fast Facts About **SUBSTANCE USE DISORDERS**: What Every Nurse, APRN, and PA Needs to Know *(Marshall, Spencer)*

Fast Facts for the **TRAVEL NURSE**: Travel Nursing *(Landrum)*

Fast Facts for the **TRIAGE NURSE**: An Orientation and Care Guide, Second Edition *(Visser, Montejano)*

Fast Facts for **WOUND CARE NURSING**: Practical Wound Management, Second Edition *(Myers)*

Fast Facts for **WRITING THE DNP PROJECT**: Effective Structure, Content, and Presentation *(Christenbery)*

Forthcoming FAST FACTS Books

Fast Facts for the **ADULT-GERONTOLOGY ACUTE CARE NURSE PRACTITIONER** *(Carpenter)*

Fast Facts About **DIVERSITY, EQUITY, AND INCLUSION** *(Davis)*

Fast Facts for the **L&D NURSE**: Labor & Delivery Orientation, Third Edition *(Groll)*

Fast Facts About **LGBTQ CARE FOR NURSES** *(Traister)*

Fast Facts for **PATIENT SAFETY IN NURSING** *(Hunt)*

Visit www.springerpub.com to order.

FAST FACTS for
WOUND CARE NURSING

Trisha Myers, MSN, APRN, FNP-BC, is a Board-Certified Nurse Practitioner at Burn and Reconstructive Centers of America. A certified wound specialist, Ms. Myers has spent more than two decades providing specialized wound care for patients with burn injuries as well as a myriad of acute, chronic, and complex wounds. She helped develop an inpatient wound consultancy program for her practice and regularly publishes articles related to burn and wound care in various scholastic journals. In the past, Ms. Myers has worked in trauma and flight nursing.

Ms. Myers graduated from the University of Nebraska in 1990 with a bachelor's degree in nursing and went on to complete a master's degree as a family nurse practitioner at Georgia Southern University in 2006.

Ms. Myers is passionate about animal welfare and is a volunteer at her local Humane Society aiding with dog rescue and rehabilitation.

FAST FACTS for
WOUND CARE NURSING

Practical Wound Management

Second Edition

Trisha Myers, MSN, APRN, FNP-BC

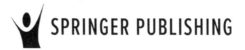

SPRINGER PUBLISHING

Springer Publishing Company, LLC
11 West 42nd Street, New York, NY 10036
www.springerpub.com
connect.springerpub.com/

Acquisitions Editor: Rachel X. Landes
Compositor: Amnet Systems

ISBN: 978-0-8261-9502-9
ebook ISBN: 978-0-8261-9509-8
DOI: 10.1891/9780826195098

21 22 23 24 / 5 4 3 2 1

Library of Congress Cataloging-in-Publication Data

I dedicate this book to the late
Dr. Joseph M. Still, whose commitment to and compassion for
burn victims and their families are unparalleled.
He was a true visionary in the field of complex wound care.

Contents

Section IV **LEGAL ASPECTS AND REGULATIONS**

Foreword

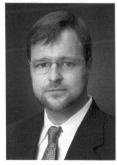

Robert F. Mullins, MD

Wounds are defined as a breakdown in the protective function of the skin or a loss of epithelial continuity following an injury. They can be described in many ways based on etiology, location, or whether they are acute or chronic in nature. What is true to any individual who cares for this entity is the impact the disease process has on the individual physically and emotionally. Approximately 15% of Medicare beneficiaries (8.2 million people) are impacted by chronic nonhealing wounds. Unfortunately, this number will only continue to grow with the aging baby boomer population and the continued lengthening of our life expectancies due to advances in modern medicine. Conservatively, the treatment of all wounds costs Medicare approximately $28–$32 billion annually. While that is a staggering number, the cost to an individual, I believe, is far greater secondary to a general loss of independence and productivity, thus summating in a nonquantifiable emotional toll.

Fortunately, there are significant advances being made in our ability to treat this disease entity through minimally invasive vascular techniques, new skin substitutes, and modulation of the healing process. However, one of the greatest advances has been made in classifying this disease process as largely preventable, thereby shifting the emphasis of healthcare providers on preventing versus treating the complication of immobility (pressure), vascular insufficiency, and/or metabolic derangements.

While techniques and products will continue to advance in the care of this patient population, we should not forget the importance of the individuals who have dedicated their lives to this patient population. I was fortunate enough to work with such an individual, Robert Fredrick "Fred" Mullins, a true pioneer and gentleman to this particular patient population. Dr. Mullins, a general surgeon, sought advanced training in burn care under the mentorship of Dr. Joseph M. Still in Augusta, Georgia. Both became well known nationally for their care of the thermally injured patient, but few knew the lives impacted by their dedication to wound patients residing in the southeastern United States. A kind soul, Dr. Mullins dedicated his life to caring for disease entities that were not easy to treat but were the ones that lacked a knowledgeable, compassionate physician. Over the years, Dr. Mullins treated thousands of wound patients referred across the Southeast but saw the need for expanded care for this patient population. In a short time, he established Burn and Advanced Wound Care Centers across the United States that offer state-of-the-art care regardless of the ability to pay for the services.

I encourage those about to read this book to absorb the knowledge found within these chapters. Once educated in advanced wound care, seek out this unique patient population and provide the emotional and physical care that they desire. In doing so, we can all join this group of compassionate healthcare providers and continue in the footsteps of Dr. Mullins by providing excellent care.

Shawn Fagan, MD, FACS
Chief Medical Officer
Burn and Reconstructive Centers
of America
Augusta, Georgia

Preface

Wounds—what a broad term! *The Original Roget's International Thesaurus* gives all of the following terms for *wounds*: *trauma, injury, hurt, lesion, cut, incision, scratch, gash, puncture, stab, laceration, mutilation, abrasion, gangrene, necrosis,* and more. If Roget were a healthcare provider looking at a wound for the first time, he would not stop with just a simple surface term. In a split second, he would send all that information to his mental search engine for processing. His simple surface term, for example, *abrasion*, would generate more sensory input, such as classification (common, complex, or atypical, chronic, or acute) and bioburden (clean, dirty, or infected). Before heaving a big sigh, he would have contemplated nutrition and pain management. After all this was sufficiently processed, another broad concept would surface. "I need a remedy." Roget's brain interface system would go into overdrive, bouncing from one neuron to another as more definitions came to mind, such as relief, help, restorative, medicine, drug, soothing, debridement, salve, antibiotics, poultices, bandage, healing, curative, restorative, palliative, protective… oh, and coming up for air… preventive. Whew!

Before your brain dendrites recoil, let me remind you of this: I am a board-certified family nurse practitioner and a wound care specialist. My goal is to simplify the wound care process for you. The wound care information in this book was written in the *Fast Facts* format to give you, the reader, access to specific information regarding the scope of wound care. The book is user-friendly and nonintimidating, making it a "must-read" for healthcare providers with a passion for pursuing the specialty of wound care.

We have come a long way since the old "barber pole" days and wet-to-dry dressings. Not only has the treatment for wounds become complex, but so have the legal aspects of wound care. It is no surprise that wound care has grown into its own specialty. This book will cut out the wordy textbook style and simplify and reinforce knowledge for the healthcare provider dedicated to providing ideal wound care in the most cost-efficient way possible. The book will also be an ideal reference guide, no matter your level of wound care interest, educational preparation, or even years of work experience. The book is designed to be an easy read, bullet-pointed with practical information. Each chapter includes a brief introduction and a feature entitled "Fast Facts" that provides insight to important wound care principles for your consideration. I encourage you to take notes and enjoy your wound care discoveries.

Best Regards!
Tish Myers

Acknowledgments

This book would not have been possible were it not for the spectrum of wound care professionals whom I have had the honor of working with, and learning from, for the last 25 years. I began my career in wound care as a nurse in a highly specialized regional burn center. I really loved taking care of these patients and had great admiration for the seasoned "burn nurses" who had made burn nursing their lifelong passion. Over the years, I worked side by side with them in the trenches, taking care of thousands of burn patients.

My journey would not have been possible without the guidance and kindness bestowed on me by the late Dr. Joseph M. Still. His vision to serve burn patients began in 1978 when he opened the Joseph M. Still Burn Center in Augusta, Georgia. Today, the center is named Burn and Reconstructive Centers of America and has become the world's leading burn treatment facility with centers across the United States.

I would like to thank and acknowledge all my colleagues throughout the years who have been instrumental in helping me grow professionally. Every one of them has helped me grow in some way or another.

Special thanks go to the team of fantastic physicians and mid-level providers whom I work with every day. Their wisdom and knowledge of wound care has shaped me into the competent clinician I am today. I would be remiss if i did not especially express gratitude to the late Dr. Robert F. Mullins for his diligent teaching and guidance of our entire team and for growing Burn and Reconstructive Centers of America into what it is today.

I would also like to thank my editor, Rachel Landes, for her expertise in helping develop this book.

And of course, thank you, my readers, for taking an interest in my book and trusting me to be your teacher. I hope you find this book to be of benefit and that the content provided within will facilitate your individual growth as a wound care specialist.

1

Defining the Spectrum of Wounds

1

Attacking the Basics: What Fuels a Wound

INTRODUCTION

Simply put, three major components control the existence and outcome of a wound:

1. *The wound environment, which ultimately is the patient.*
2. *The healthcare providers and the caretakers.*
3. *The type of dressing.*

Each of these components has both intrinsic and extrinsic factors that play a role in whether an acceptable or positive outcome is achieved. The ability to change these factors ultimately influences the outcome, as it pertains to the realistic time frame and ability to heal a wound. As Confucius said, "By nature, men are nearly alike; by practice, they get to be wide apart." The same is true of wounds; no two are exactly alike. This chapter will help you understand what fuels a wound and how to start your approach in wound care and wound healing.

In this chapter, you will learn:

1. The three major components that contribute to optimal wound healing and the extrinsic and intrinsic factors that influence them.

2. How the wound care provider works in conjunction with other specialists, staff, and family members to provide and manage personalized wound care plans and to educate and empower novice staff, patients, and caretakers.

MAJOR COMPONENT 1: THE PATIENT AND THE PHYSIOLOGIC ENVIRONMENT

To understand what fuels a wound, the healthcare provider must understand the wound from the inside out. This knowledge will come from knowing what intrinsic and extrinsic factors are driving the wound. Obtaining a thorough and accurate history and assessment of the patient is the initial step. Take the time to know your patient.

Extrinsic patient factors to note:

- For the history
  - Lifestyle factors such as smoking and use of alcohol
  - Socioeconomic status
- For assessment
  - Moisture
  - Mechanical stress such as compression, tension, shear, or contractures
  - Chemical stress such as what occurs when tissue is damaged or inflamed
  - Infection

Intrinsic patient factors to note:

- Age
- Comorbidities
- Diabetes
- Peripheral vascular disease
- Chronic cardiopulmonary disease
- Cardiovascular disease
- Obesity
- Autoimmune disorders
- Nutritional status
- Overall health and well-being

LIFESTYLE FACTORS

Nicotine is a potent vasoconstrictor; it reduces the flow of vital nutrients and oxygen to tissue. Nicotine also increases platelet adhesiveness, resulting in microvascular occlusion, and reduces proliferation of red blood cells. Both carbon monoxide and cyanide inhibit oxygen transport to cells and interfere with cellular metabolism.

Excessive alcohol intake impairs wound healing by compromising the immune system, therefore increasing the likelihood of infections, and by increasing the risk of bleeding. People who drink alcohol in excess are concomitantly malnourished.

Patients with a wound of any nature must be counseled on the importance of smoking cessation and limiting alcohol intake. Incorporate assistive aids and resources into the patients' plan of care to facilitate these lifestyle modifications.

MOISTURE

Maceration caused by incontinence, sweating, or excess exudate from a wound bed all contribute to the breakdown of tissue. Consider the patient's ability to manage continence and intervene as warranted, especially for patients with mobility and sensory limitations.

Interventions to manage incontinence:

- Incontinence briefs
- Indwelling urinary catheters
- Condom catheters for men
- Purewick urine collection systems for women
- Fecal diversion with colostomies

Be diligent in managing both urinary and fecal incontinence and protect the incontinent patient's skin from prolonged contact with urine and feces with barrier products.

Barrier products:

- Calmoseptine
- Petroleum jelly
- Zinc oxide

Ensure the wound bed is free of excessive moisture, particularly by managing exudate with the appropriate type of dressing. Selecting correct dressings is discussed in detail in Chapter 9.

MECHANICAL STRESS

Tissue ischemia and eventual breakdown occur when a patient is immobile and pressure is exerted over bony prominences. Tissue damage can occur within 15 minutes of diminished blood flow. The forces of shearing and friction occur when the tissues underneath the skin are forced to move, such as when pulling instead of lifting a patient when the patient is lying down or sitting. Extremity contractures also cause mechanical stress by causing tissue ischemia.

Breakdown due to mechanical stress can best be prevented by frequent and diligent repositioning, by use of pressure-relieving devices, and by placing pillows between pressure areas such as the knees.

Pressure-relieving devices:

- Low-air-loss mattresses
- Heel and elbow protectors
- Prevalon boots
- Rojo cushions

CHEMICAL STRESS

If used in excess, common over-the-counter antiseptics and cleaning agents such as iodine, hydrogen peroxide, and rubbing alcohol can damage healthy cells. While they may reduce the bacterial load on the surface of a wound, they have no real effect below the skin's surface. Most wounds can be cleaned with simple soap and water. However, a number of wound cleaning solutions are available from companies that specialize in wound products that are not harmful to healing wounds.

INFECTIONS AND BIOBURDENS

Two of the most important components influencing wound healing are infection and bioburden. An *infection* occurs when pathogens colonize to the point of invading the host tissue. Pathogens can originate from several environmental sources that harbor bacteria, viruses, and fungus. Skin, in a healthy state, protects the body from invasion of pathogens through its stratum corneum layer. Additional body defenses against the invasion of pathogens include secretions from sebaceous glands and the body's immune system. Some pathogens are part of the body's natural flora and become harmful only after invading the tissue. These opportunistic pathogens are so named because they attack the body's defenses when an opportunity presents itself, such as during surgery, in the event of trauma, or through an existing wound. *Bioburden* is the number of contaminating pathogens on the surface of a wound.

Contamination is the presence of pathogens on the surface of the skin or a wound. *Colonization* occurs when contaminants multiply significantly and the body's immune system is overwhelmed. Signs of inflammation become apparent: redness, heat, and/or drainage.

BIOFILMS

A *biofilm* is the extracellular matrix structure that attaches itself to a wound's surface tissue and protects pathogens from the host's defenses. Literature suggests that 60% to 90% of chronic wounds contain biofilm-forming bacteria.

A biofilm structure attaches itself firmly to the surrounding surface of the wound and must be scrubbed off; simply spritzing wound cleanser or pouring sterile water on the wound is not effective. Chronic wound biofilms tend to be highly resistant to antimicrobial agents.

Common biofilm-forming bacteria:

- *Staphylococcus aureus* (staph)
- *Pseudomonas aeruginosa*
- *Beta-haemolytic streptococci* (Strep)
- *Enterococcus*
- *Klebsiella pneumoniae*
- *Acinetobacter*
- *Enterobacter*
- *Candida* (yeast)

Factors that lead from wound contamination to biofilm to infection include:

- Pathogens resistant to antibiotic therapy
- The type and variety of pathogens
- The interaction of different bacterial species with each other
- The host's immune system response

Some of the most recent alternative treatments developed to target biofilms include:

- Negative pressure wound therapy (a mainstay of wound care)
- Blue light therapy
- Nano-antimicrobial agents embedded or coated onto dressings and drains
    - Silver, copper, and zinc
- Modulation of pH with agents
    - Acetic acid 1% or 5%, ascorbic acid, Medihoney
- Medical maggots
- Hyperbaric oxygen therapy
- Surfactant-based products
    - Plurogel, Aquacel Ag, Hydrogel, and Silvasorb gel
- Probiotics

Wound Agents
Bactericidal: An agent that destroys bacteria.
Bacteriostatic: An agent that can prevent new bacteria from growing or multiplying without destroying bacteria that are already present.

DIAGNOSTIC FOLLOW-UP FOR CONFIRMING WOUND INFECTION

Tissue biopsies, needle aspiration, and swab samples are the most common lab tests for diagnosing an infection. All chronic wounds are contaminated; therefore, diagnose actual wound infection based on clinical signs and from culture results. The goal is to establish a host-manageable bioburden.

Tissue Biopsies

Tissue biopsies can be completed utilizing a simple punch biopsy at the bedside or during surgical debridement. If osteomyelitis is suspected, it will be necessary for the provider to obtain a bone biopsy. While most bone biopsies are usually collected during surgical debridement, the procedure can be done at the bedside on select patients.

Clinical Indications for a Wound Culture
- Systemic signs of infection, fever, leukocytosis (i.e., elevated white blood cell count)
- **Sudden high blood glucose**
- **Increasing pain in a neuropathic extremity**
- **Lack of healing of a clean-appearing wound after 2 weeks**

Signs and Symptoms of Infection at the Wound Site
- Pain or tenderness
- Excess drainage
- Red color
- Cutaneous warmth
- Unusual or foul odor
- Swelling or firmness (induration)

Needle Aspiration

In needle aspiration, a thin needle is inserted directly into tissue; cells are aspirated and sent to pathology or microbiology for identification.

Swab Samples

A swab culture is taken by swabbing the surface of a wound or within the cavity of a wound. Exudate can also be collected by a swab culture. Swab cultures can easily be contaminated during the collection process, so be diligent with the collection process.

The Levine technique is believed to be most reflective of tissue bioburden. Rotate a swab over a 1 cm² area with sufficient pressure to express fluid from within the wound tissue.

TREATMENT OF INFECTIONS

Treatment is targeted at reducing a wound's bacterial load and biofilm. The most effective treatment plan is combination therapy consisting of appropriate antibiotic selection based on culture sensitivities and dressing selection. See Tables 1.1 and 1.2.

Antimicrobial topical ointment and creams include:

- Bacitracin or Polysporin: Effective only against bacterial infections
- Bactroban 2%: Effective primarily against Gram-positive bacteria Staph and Strep including methicillin-resistant *S. aureus* (MRSA)
- Silver sulfadiazine cream 1%
- Sulfamylon cream 5%

SOCIOECONOMIC STATUS

When establishing a wound care treatment plan, consider the patient's ability to afford the medications and products being prescribed and the ability to correctly carry out the wound care treatment. Many antibiotics, wound care products, and dressing supplies can be expensive and complicated to administer. Always determine if the patient's insurance provider will cover the products being prescribed. The treatment plan may have to be adjusted if the payor source will not cover certain products or if the patient is uninsured.

Provide extensive and ongoing education and demonstration to whomever will be performing the wound care treatments to ensure understanding and the ability to complete the task. Failure to address

Table 1.1

Antimicrobial Topical Solutions

Solution	Effectiveness
Dakin's solution (sodium hypochlorite)	Broad-spectrum; effective against MRSA, VRE, other bacteria, viruses, mold, fungi, and yeast.
Puracyn Plus (hypochlorous acid)	The same molecule that the body's neutrophils create as part of the immune system. Provides broad-spectrum coverage.
Silver nitrate 0.5% solution	Broad-spectrum bacteriostatic effective against many Gram-positive and Gram-negative bacteria.
Sulfamylon/mafenide acetate	Effective against systemic fungal infections and can be mixed with Amphotericin B.

MRSA, methicillin-resistant *Staphylococcus aureus*; VRE, vancomycin-resistant enterococci.

Table 1.2

Antimicrobial Topical Dressings

Dressing	Effectiveness
Acticoat	Broad-spectrum effectiveness.
Exsalt	Can be left intact for several days, therefore, requires fewer dressing changes.
KerraContact Ag	
Mepilex Ag	Well tolerated.
Mepitel Ag	
Promogran Prisma	
Tritec Silver Nanocrystal based	
AMD kerlix (Polyhexamethylene Biguanide)	Highly effective against most organisms.

both these factors will lead to a less than favorable outcome and noncompliance.

AGE

As we age, our skin becomes much drier and thinner as we lose secretory cells that help maintain moisture and elasticity. Teach patients and their care providers how to keep the skin well hydrated with a nonalcohol-based moisturizer.

COMORBIDITIES

Many chronic health conditions such as diabetes, chronic kidney disease, cardiopulmonary disease, cardiovascular disease, cancer, and autoimmune-driven conditions can both cause a wound to develop and impede wound healing. It is critical that patients with a wound have regular appointments with their primary care provider with the goal of optimal chronic disease management in mind.

Fast Facts

- Uncontrolled diabetes can affect wound healing by damaging nerves resulting in lack of sensation, causing poor immune system response, creating a high-risk environment for wound infection, and causing impaired blood flow.
- Smoking affects wound healing by impairing tissue oxygenation and collagen deposition necessary for wound closure.
- Pain affects wound healing by causing vasoconstriction and immune system suppression.

NUTRITION

The role of nutrition in wound care must not be overlooked. Both macronutrients and micronutrients must be in balance to provide an optimal state for wound healing. See Table 1.3. It is estimated that caloric needs during wound healing are 30–40 kcal/kg.

Macronutrients	Carbohydrates, fats, proteins, and fluids
Micronutrients	Amino acids, vitamins, and minerals

When assessing the patient with a wound, note if the patient has inadequate intake.

Causes of inadequate nutritional intake:

- Poor appetite
- Inability to feed oneself
- Overeating
- Impaired sense of taste or smell
- Difficulty swallowing

Physical assessment:

- Weight and weight loss or gain
- Body mass index

Table 1.3

Laboratory Parameters		
	Normal Ranges	**Possible Indications**
Serum albumin	3.4–5.4 g/dL	A lower level can indicate malnutrition.
Serum prealbumin	15–36 mg/dL	A lower level can indicate malnutrition.
Retinol-binding protein	40–60 ug/mL	A lower level can indicate nutritional deficiencies.
Serum creatinine	0.6–1.2 mg/dL for males 0.5–1.1 mg/dL for females	A lower level indicates too little creatine in muscle tissue.
Transferrin	170–370 mg/dL	A lower level can indicate liver disease or hemolytic anemia.

- Loss of subcutaneous fat
- Edema
- Muscle wasting
- Fatigue
- Reduced grip strength

Fluid intake is another important factor to consider. The goal for the patient with a wound is 1 mL/kcal/day but will need to be adjusted for insensible fluid losses and for patients with cardiac and renal disease.

Causes of insensible fluid loss:

- Fever
- Vomiting
- Diarrhea
- Diuresis
- Fistulae output
- Wound exudate

The patient's socioeconomic status should also be assessed since many people, particularly the elderly, have social and economic difficulties that put them at nutritional risk. Determine their access to and ability to afford food, ability to prepare food, and availability of resources.

The Mini Nutritional Assessment is a widely used tool to assess malnutrition. It incorporates food intake, weight loss patterns, mobility, and neuropsychiatric contributors to eating (see Exhibit 1.1).

Diagnostic markers to assess nutritional status:

- Albumin
- Prealbumin
- Transferrin
- C-reactive protein

It is important to establish a nutritional plan as part of the overall wound care treatment plan (see Table 1.4). Some patients may need modified diets depending on the ability to chew and swallow while others may need feeding tubes. In addition to education regarding a balanced diet, incorporate supplemental micronutrients such as arginine, glutamine, and multivitamins. The anabolic steroid oxandrolone is an effective pharmacological agent to reduce protein catabolism in patients with burn injuries and complex wounds. The recommended dose is 5 to 10 mg BID. There are many protein supplements available in various forms such as powders, shakes, and bars that can be added to the patient's diet.

MAJOR COMPONENT 2: THE HEALTHCARE PROVIDERS AND THE CARETAKERS

For the sick, it is important to have the best.

Florence Nightingale

You will not likely know what patients you will care for each day or even what wounds they will have. What is your plan? What is your goal for your patients today?

The goal of wound care specialists is to raise the bar in wound care management. Considering current healthcare and economic issues, we need now more than ever to step up and define our position. Wound care teams have the potential to save hospitals money, improve patient outcomes, and raise the "novice-to-expert" bar related to wound care in every unit with a consultancy team approach. No matter the organization or healthcare facility, a wound care provider's responsibilities and roles are threefold—clinical expert, educator, and researcher:

Clinical Expert: Directing Wound Management

- Understands the healthcare system's group purchasing organization.
- Works with the facility's purchasing staff/formulary to develop state-of-the-art wound management formularies and shared cost-reduction strategy goals.
- Shares responsibility for development and implementation of wound and skin care policies, procedures, and guidelines.

Exhibit 1.1

Mini Nutritional Assessment Tool

Mini Nutritional Assessment
MNA®

Nestlé
NutritionInstitute

Last name: _____   First name: _____

Sex: _____   Age: _____   Weight, kg: _____   Height, cm: _____   Date: _____

Complete the screen by filling in the boxes with the appropriate numbers.
Add the numbers for the screen. If score is 11 or less, continue with the assessment to gain a Malnutrition Indicator Score.

Screening

A   Has food intake declined over the past 3 months due to loss of appetite, digestive problems, chewing or swallowing difficulties?

0 = severe decrease in food intake
1 = moderate decrease in food intake
2 = no decrease in food intake   ☐

B   Weight loss during the last 3 months

0 = weight loss greater than 3kg (6.6lbs)
1 = does not know
2 = weight loss between 1 and 3kg (2.2 and 6.6 lbs)
3 = no weight loss   ☐

C   Mobility

0 = bed or chair bound
1 = able to get out of bed / chair but does not go out
2 = goes out   ☐

D   Has suffered psychological stress or acute disease in the past 3 months?

0 = yes   2 = no   ☐

J   How many full meals does the patient eat daily?

0 = 1 meal
1 = 2 meals
2 = 3 meals   ☐

K   Selected consumption markers for protein intake

• At least one serving of dairy products
 (milk, cheese, yoghurt) per day   yes ☐ no ☐
• Two or more servings of legumes
 or eggs per week   yes ☐ no ☐
• Meat, fish or poultry every day   yes ☐ no ☐

0.0 = if 0 or 1 yes
0.5 = if 2 yes
1.0 = if 3 yes   ☐☐

L   Consumes two or more servings of fruit or vegetables per day?

0 = no   1 = yes   ☐

M   How much fluid (water, juice, coffee, tea, milk...) is consumed per day?

0.0 = less than 3 cups
0.5 = 3 to 5 cups
1.0 = more than 5 cups   ☐☐

E Neuropsychological problems
0 = severe dementia or depression
1 = mild dementia
2 = no psychological problems ☐

F Body Mass Index (BMI) (weight in kg) / (height in m²)
0 = BMI less than 19
1 = BMI 19 to less than 21
2 = BMI 21 to less than 23
3 = BMI 23 or greater ☐☐

Screening score (subtotal max. 14 points)
12-14 points: Normal nutritional status
8-11 points: At risk of malnutrition
0-7 points. Malnourished

For a more in-depth assessment, continue with questions G-R

Assessment

G Lives independently (not in nursing home or hospital)
1 = yes 0 = no ☐

H Takes more than 3 prescription drugs per day
0 = yes 1 = no ☐

I Pressure sores or skin ulcers
0 = yes 1 = no ☐

N Mode of feeding
0 = unable to eat without assistance
1 = self-fed with some difficulty
2 = self-fed without any problem ☐

O Self view of nutritional status
0 = views self as being malnourished
1 = is uncertain of nutritional state
2 = views self as having no nutritional problem ☐

P In comparison with other people of the same age, how does the patient consider his / her health status?
0.0 = not as good
0.5 = does not know
1.0 = as good
2.0 = better ☐.☐

Q Mid-arm circumference (MAC) in cm
0.0 = MAC less than 21
0.5 = MAC 21 to 22
1.0 = MAC 22 or greater ☐☐

R Calf circumference (CC) in cm
0 = CC less than 31
1 = CC 31 or greater ☐

Assessment (max. 16 points) ☐☐☐
Screening score ☐☐☐
Total Assessment (max. 30 points) ☐☐☐

Malnutrition Indicator Score
24 to 30 points ☐ Normal nutritional status
17 to 23.5 points ☐ At risk of malnutrition
Less than 17 points ☐ Malnourished

References
1 Vellas B. Villars H. Abellan G. et al. Overview of the MNA® - Its History and Challenges. J Nutr Health Aging 2006; 10:456-465.
2 Rubenstein LZ. Harker JO. Salva A. Guigoz Y. Vellas B. Screening for Undernutrition in Geriatric Practice: Developing the Short-Form Mini Nutritional Assessment (MNA-SF). J Geront 2001; 56A: M366-377
3 Guigoz Y. The Mini-Nutritional Assessment (MNA®) Review of the Literature - What does it tell us? J Nutr Health Aging 2006; 10:466-487.

Source: From Société Des Produits Nestlé S.A. 1994, Revision 2009.

Chapter 1 Attacking the Basics: What Fuels a Wound

Table 1.4

The Importance of Nutrition

The Six Major Classes of Nutrients	Role in the Wound Healing Process	Calorie % Needed for Daily Allowance
Carbohydrates	Provide energy and prevent gluconeogenesis.	50%–60%
Proteins/amino acids	Repair and synthesize enzymes, collagen, and connective tissue. Also aid cell multiplication and production of antibodies.	20%–25%
Fats/fatty acids	Stored triglycerides are concentrated sources and reserves of energy.	20%–25%
Vitamins	Vitamin C is essential for collagen synthesis.	60 mg daily
	Vitamin A helps epithelialization, wound closure, and inflammatory response and counteracts delayed healing in patients on corticosteroids.	25,000 IU daily for 10 days if on high doses of steroids
Minerals	Copper aids the cross-linking of collagen.	900 mcg daily
	Iron aids collagen formation.	8 mg daily
	Magnesium promotes protein synthesis.	350 mg daily
	Zinc aids collagen formation, protein synthesis, blood clotting, and immune system function.	200–300 mg daily
Water	Aids in hydration and oxygen perfusion. Also acts as a solvent for small molecules such as minerals, vitamins, amino acids, and glucose moving in and out of cell walls.	Patients on air-fluidized beds require an additional 500 mL of fluid daily.

Educator: Empowering Staff by Teaching

- Is able and willing to train students and new providers and to offer novice staff wound care support.
- Develops a program for organizing wound and skin care products.
- Teaches the program and products to the wound care team and staff.
- Understands that wound care can be intimidating, continually changing, and frustrating to staff. The wound care provider is the resource for problem-solving, the sounding board, and the wound care escalation point person.

Researcher: Improving Quality, Making Evaluations, and Collecting Data

- Understands the scope of studies and appraises quality improvement.
- Understands and develops clinical markers for treatment options and guidelines–from aggressive wound care to palliative care.
- Observes the wound team members and helps develop novice team members to consultancy experts or providers who can empower others.

Even the best wound care providers will experience a less-than-desired outcome for their patients if the caretakers are unwilling or unable to implement the treatment plan effectively. The wound care provider and team must carefully assess who will be the patients' primary care providers and ensure ongoing education and hands-on instruction pertaining to wound care, dressing changes, pressure redistribution, incontinence management, nutrition, and so forth.

In this case, enlist the assistance from community resources such as home health to include skilled nurses and aides, physical and occupational therapists, and respite or hospice services as needed. If the patient will be placed in an acute care facility or long-term skilled nursing facility, determine if the facility has the resources necessary to treat a patient with a complex wound.

When considering a new facility, consider the following:

- Does the facility have a dedicated wound care nurse or team?
- Can they get the wound care supplies necessary to manage the wound appropriately?
- Can they provide regular follow-up with the wound care health provider?

MAJOR COMPONENT 3: TYPE OF DRESSING

Wound care dressings can be complex, so make good choices for each individual wound. Wound care specialists must stay abreast of manufacturers and the latest technologies in wound care offerings. Get to know your wound care representatives. Ask for samples, open the products, and examine them and compare them with others in the same category. Ask questions to determine what characteristics of individual products make them preferable and find out how they will benefit your patients' wounds. Patients and their care providers can also provide invaluable information regarding types of wound dressings and products, so ask questions with every visit. Important information to gather includes ease of use and administration, comfort/pain, and affordability. Selecting the correct dressings and the types of dressings will be discussed at length in Chapter 9.

Fast Facts

Question: How do you know that a wound care product is what it claims to be?

Answer: The U.S. FDA establishes and monitors the quality of dressings and products and addresses violations from manufacturers, which is detailed on 510 (k) forms. Wound care providers should determine if the products they are using are FDA approved.

Bibliography

Kadam, S., Shai, S., Shahane, A., & Kaushik, K. (2019, April 30). Recent advances in non-conventional antimicrobial approaches for chronic wound biofilms: Have we found the "chink in the armor"? *Biomedicines, 7*(2), 2–13. Retrieved from https://www.ncbi.nlm.nih.gov

Nestle HealthScience Mini Nutritional Assessment. Retrieved from www.mna-elderly.com

Quain, A., & Khardori, N. (2015, December). Nutrition in wound care management: A comprehensive overview. *Wounds, 27*(12), 2–4. Retrieved from https://www.ncbi.nlm.nih.gov

Rehm, K. (2015, December). Exploring options for certification in wound care. *9*(9), 2. Retrieved from https://www.TodaysWoundClinic.com

2

The Phases of Wound Healing and Types of Wound Closure

INTRODUCTION

> Do as much as possible for the patient, and a little as possible to the patient.
>
> —*Dr. Bernard Lown*

This chapter is about becoming proficient in understanding skin structure and function, understanding the normal wound healing process, and knowing the factors that influence this process. The goal for the wound care practitioner is to optimize the healing process, maximize functional performance, and improve the quality of life for the patient whenever possible.

In this chapter, you will learn:

1. The structure and function of skin.
2. The three phases of wound healing and types of scar tissue.

THE STRUCTURE AND FUNCTION OF SKIN

Knowing the structure and function of the skin and their correlation to the different types of wounds and wound healing is essential. The skin is the largest organ, encompassing the greatest amount of body surface area. As Figure 2.1 describes, the skin consists of three distinct layers: the epidermis, dermis, and hypodermis or subcutaneous layer. The primary function of skin is to act as a barrier from pathogens and to help regulate body temperature through sweating and changes in peripheral circulation. Skin also acts as a repository for Vitamin D and as a sensory organ due to an extensive network of nerve cells that detect changes in environmental stimuli.

The epidermis is the outer layer of the skin and is composed mostly of keratinocytes, which are the protein building blocks. The epidermis is avascular and, therefore, dependent on the dermis for delivery of nutrients. Its primary function is to act as a barrier to the external environment. The epidermis also contains melanocytes, which are responsible for the pigmentation or color of the skin and for absorbing ultraviolet radiation from the sun.

The dermis forms the inner layer and is much thicker than the epidermis. Collagen and elastin are the major components of the dermis and are responsible for the skin's strength and elasticity. The primary functions include protection by cushioning the deeper layers from injury and nourishment of the epidermis. In terms of wound healing, the dermis holds mast cells responsible for controlling immune and inflammatory responses. The dermis also

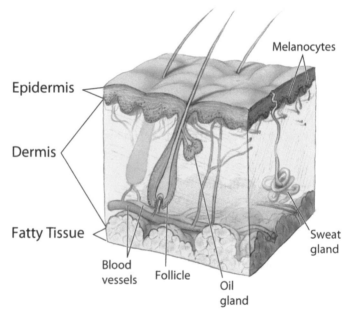

Figure 2.1 The structure of the skin.
Source: WebMD, LLC.

contains a vast network of blood vessels, nerve fibers, hair follicles, sweat glands, and oil glands.

The hypodermis, also known as the subcutaneous layer, lies below the dermis and is comprised mostly of fat. It insulates and absorbs trauma.

THE THREE PHASES OF CHRONIC WOUND HEALING

Inflammatory Phase

- Characterized by the cleaning of the wound.
- Involves inflammatory cells: neutrophils, macrophages, and lymphocytes.
- All three types of inflammatory cells destroy bacteria via vasodilation and phagocytosis.
- Macrophages come from monocytes, which provide growth factors and cytokines, which are immunomodulating agents.
- Duration: Averages 2 to 5 days
- Signs and symptoms: Discomfort, mild wound periphery redness, and swelling

Proliferation Phase

- Characterized by tissue granulation
  - Typically, this is when 50% or more of the wound is granulating and contracting inward
- Involves proteoglycans, fibroblasts, collagen, and glycosaminoglycans that fill the wound bed and produce new capillaries through angiogenesis.
- Duration: 2 days to 3 weeks or more depending on the size and type of wound
- Signs and symptoms:
  - Production of granulation (beefy red tissue that easily bleeds).
  - Wound contraction (getting smaller from the edges inward).
  - Epithelialization (wound being covered by skin).

Remodeling Phase

- Characterized by the formation of new collagen, which is required for tensile strength and, eventually, scar formation.
- Duration: 3 weeks to 2 years
- Signs and symptoms: This collagen deposition and remodeling cause the new skin (scar tissue) to reach a tensile strength of approximately 80%.

How to tell the difference between granulation tissue and epithelium

- Healthy granulation tissue is beefy red, shiny, and bumpy. It bleeds easily.
- New epithelium changes from a shiny, granulated look to a polished pink sheen as blood vessels heal and are not needed in the formation of scar tissue.
- A wound may look as if it has healed but may require time for collagen deposition to reach the tensile strength of scar tissue, which is required to resist breakdown.

THREE TYPES OF WOUND CLOSURE

Primary Intention

These are wounds that are closed, or approximated, with sutures, staples, glue, or Steri-Strips. Examples include surgical wounds and lacerations.

Secondary Intention

These wounds heal by granulation and contraction. An example is a chronic wound such as a pressure injury.

Tertiary Intention (Delayed Primary)

These are wounds that are purposely kept open for observation and treatment of contamination, draining, cleaning, and debridement if necessary. Typically, tertiary intention wounds are surgical wounds and are generally closed later.

An example is a dehisced or eviscerated abdominal wound.

TYPES OF SCAR TISSUE

Hypertrophic Scars

These scars extend above the surrounding skin. They can be discolored but usually fade with time.

Keloid Scars

These scars are fibrous, ridged, and raised and can be painful or itchy. Keloids are considered benign tumors (never malignant). People who have darkly pigmented skin are more prone to develop keloid scar tissue than people with lighter skin pigmentation.

Treatment options for keloids include foam dressings, silicone gel pads, compression garments, cortisone injections, and laser therapy.

Contractures

Contractures are proliferations of scar tissue and normal tissue that draw up and pull and are often seen with healing burn injuries. Contractures affect joint mobility, sometimes to the extent of severely reducing joint flexibility.

Treatment options include aggressive occupational and physical therapy, splinting, specific positioning, and often, surgical release of the scar tissue.

Fast Facts

Physiology of Fetal Wound Healing

- Fetal skin can heal without scar formation, but there is still much to learn about the process, which is related to biomedical ethics.
- The amniotic fluid may contribute to wound healing, which is rich in hyaluronic acid, fibronectin, and growth factors.
- Hyaluronic acid is a key component of the extracellular matrix and promotes cellular proliferation, tissue regeneration, and repair.
- Hyalomatrix, a wound care product composed of hyaluronic acid, is available for use today.

Bibliography

Lawton, S. (2019, November 25). Skin 1: The structure and functions of the skin. *Nursing Times (online), 115*(12), 30–33. Retrieved from https.www.nursingtimes.net

Chapter 2   The Phases of Wound Healing and Types of Wound Closure

3

Acute Wounds

INTRODUCTION

Acute wounds begin with an injury to the skin that causes bleeding, triggers clot formation, and results in the wound healing cascade. Acute wounds occur because of sudden injury or trauma and usually cause a superficial skin injury or partial-thickness wound that heals as expected according to the normal healing process via primary or secondary intention. Examples of acute wounds include lacerations, abrasions, contusions, hematomas, skin tears, and burns. Wounds that occur as a direct result of surgery are also considered acute wounds and, in some instances, may have delayed closure, as in the case of dehisced surgical abdominal wounds.

In this chapter, you will learn:

1. The types of and treatment for superficial skin injuries.
2. How to classify and care for skin tears.
3. How to determine depth of a burn and total body surface area.
4. How to treat a burn injury or when to refer.

SUPERFICIAL SKIN INJURIES

Superficial skin injuries are wounds not related to pressure, chronic disease such as diabetes, peripheral vascular disease, or autoimmune disorders. They are not documented under the National Pressure

Injury Advisory Panel (NPIAP) and are not staged. Superficial skin injuries are defined as superficial or partial-thickness wounds and are usually related to minor injuries, trauma, bites, or punctures.

Abrasions

Also known as scrapes or scratches, abrasions are a type or superficial skin injury that involve loss of patches of epidermis or superficial cutting or slicing that does not penetrate the dermis. Treatment consists of gentle cleaning of the wound with soap and water or wound cleanser and applying antimicrobial ointments such as Bacitracin, Polysporin, or Neosporin once or twice a day and covering with a simple dressing such as an adhesive bandage or other nonstick product. These wounds generally heal without complications in a matter of days.

Bruises

Also called contusions, bruises are caused from a direct blow or other injury that damages the blood vessels causing bleeding into the dermis. Very little treatment is necessary for bruises, although cold compresses can help with discomfort and swelling. Sometimes extensive bruises, such as those that occur from trauma, can evolve into a hematoma.

An area of tissue with a hematoma will feel firm (indurated) and can be quite painful. Careful assessment for the development of infection is warranted by the healthcare provider, and antibiotics may be necessary if the site becomes reddened or hot to the touch. Compression bandages such as Ace wraps can assist with resorption of a hematoma.

Lacerations

Lacerations are cuts that extend into the dermal layers and often require closure with sutures or staples. Depending on the nature and location of the laceration, antibiotics may be required as some of these acute-type injuries can be very dirty.

Fast Facts

Recommended Tetanus Booster Protocol
Minor, clean wounds: Obtain booster within 72 hours. Booster needed every 10 years.

Dirty wounds: Obtain booster within 24 hours. Booster needed per age recommendation protocol.

Skin Tears

A skin tear is a wound resulting from trauma that causes separation of the epidermis from the dermis. Depending on the severity of the friction and/or shearing forces, the tear can be simple or severe, the latter consisting of flap loss, hematoma, and tissue death.

Skin tears are classified according to tissue loss. Document if a skin tear is present on first assessment of the patient or if it is acquired while in a hospital or other facility. Documentation should include pain level, date the injury occurred, cause of the skin tear, location, size, and wound classification. Do not "stage" skin tears as they are not related to pressure.

Treatment for skin tears:

- Gently cleanse with soap and water or wound cleanser.
- Irrigate the remaining flap and pat dry.
- Apply pressure if needed to stop bleeding.
- Reposition and approximate the remaining flap.
- Choose the dressing based on the wound and drainage.
  - Several optimal dressing choices include silicone face foams, Allevyn, Mepilex, or hydrogel sheets.
- Do not apply tension when applying the dressing.
- Place a mark or arrow on the dressing to indicate the direction of the flap.
  - The arrow will indicate to the caretaker what direction to remove the dressing to avoid pulling off the fragile flap.
- Optimal secondary dressings can be used if necessary.
  - Optimal choices include tubular support dressings such as SePro Net and Spandage.

The Payne-Martin Classification for Skin Tears

Category 1: The entire epidermal flap can be approximated; there is no tissue loss.
- **A.** *Linear type:* The epidermis and dermis are pulled in one layer from the supporting structure.
- **B.** *Flat type:* The epidermis and dermis are separated, but the epidermal flap can be approximated to within 1 mm of the wound margins.

Category 2: There is partial tissue loss of the flap.
- **A.** Less than 25% of the epidermal flap is lost.
- **B.** More than 25% of the epidermal flap is lost.

Category 3: There is complete tissue loss of the flap.

Care and prevention of skin tears include educating the patient, family, and caretaker regarding frequent application of moisturizers, hydration, and protection alternatives.

- When choosing moisturizers, opt for pH-balanced, alcohol-free products that contain silicones, if possible.
- If the patient is ambulatory, suggest they apply moisturizer three or four times a day.
- The caretaker may choose to remoisturize the patient to coincide with the repositioning schedule.
- Use a lift sheet to move and/or turn the patient gently.
- Pad bedrails, wheelchair arms, and any other surfaces with which skin can make contact.
- Use pillows or blankets to provide support and prevent the patient from dangling the arms and legs.

Common Errors in Documentation

Three of the most common skin injuries that are confused in documentation are contact dermatitis, incontinence dermatitis, and candidiasis.

Contact Dermatitis

- Occurs when skin comes into contact with an irritant such as soap, cosmetics, lotions, detergents, or environmental sources such as poison ivy.
- Symptoms include a rash at the site of contact with severe itching.
- Treatment consists of cortisone ointments.

Incontinence Dermatitis

- Presents as reddened irritation or erosion of the buttocks and perineum from exposure to urine and stool and may progress to vesicular blisters.
- Treatment consists of barrier ointments such as zinc oxide and Calmoseptine, as well as frequent changes of incontinence briefs and judicious peri-care.

Candidiasis

- Presents as a red, pustular fungal rash with or without satellite lesions. Most commonly occurs in warm, moist areas such as skin folds and may have a bad odor with "cottage cheese" appearing buildup.
- Treatment consists of antifungal ointments or creams such as Clotrimazole or Miconazole, as well as keeping skin folds clean and dry.

BURNS

Burn injuries can range from a mild sunburn to a large body surface area full-thickness burn. See Table 3.1. Early stabilization and resuscitation greatly influences a burn patient's outcome. The depth and size of a burn, the part(s) of the body burned, whether smoke inhalation is present, and the patient's age and overall health can all affect the outcome.

Table 3.1

Depth of Burns	
Degree	**Description**
Superficial partial thickness (first degree)	Red, intact epidermis that blanches and is painful. Not associated with blisters or epidermal sloughing, such as a sunburn.
Partial thickness (second degree)	Blisters with epidermal sloughing. Dermis appears pink or red, moist, and blanches. Deep partial-thickness burns will appear more cherry red and dry and blanche poorly. These burns are very painful as the nerve endings are exposed.
Full thickness (third degree)	Brown or white in appearance with eschar, very dry, do not blanche. These areas of burn are painless.
Deep full thickness (fourth degree)	Charred appearance with tissue damage that involves the muscle, tendons, and bone. These areas of burn are also painless.

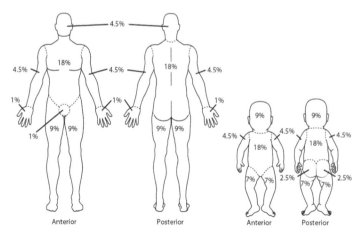

Figure 3.1 Rule of nines burn chart.

Source: Reproduced from Veenema, T. G. (2019). *Disaster nursing and emergency preparedness: For chemical, biological, and radiological terrorism and other hazards* (4th ed.) Springer Publishing Company.

Causes of Burn Injuries

- Thermal contact (such as scalding, flame, or flash)
- Frostbite
- Friction (road rash)
- Chemical contact (acids or bases)
- Electrical contact (including lightning)
- Radiation
- Inhalation with injury above or below the glottis

It is vital to know the nearest burn center and be familiar with criteria for transfer to a burn center.

Total Body Surface Area

In addition to knowing the depth of the burn, know the extent of the burn by calculating the total body surface area (TBSA). There are two formulas to calculate TBSA which include:

1. The Lund-Browder diagram, or the rule of nines (see Figure 3.1).
2. Rule of palm (the patient's palm = 1% of body surface area).

Burn Center Referral Criteria

The American Burn Association has established the following criteria for referral to a burn center:

- Partial-thickness burns greater than 10% TBSA in any age group
- Third-degree burns in any age group
- Burns that involve the face, hands, feet, genitalia, perineum, or major joints
- Any type of chemical burns
- Electrical burns, including injury by lightning strike
- Smoke inhalation injury
- Patients with burns and concomitant trauma in which the burn poses the greatest risk of morbidity and mortality
- Burn injury in patients who will require special emotional, social, or rehabilitative intervention
- Burned children in hospitals without qualified personnel or equipment for the care of children
- Burns in patients with pre-existing medical disorders that could complicate management, prolong recovery, or affect mortality

Fast Facts

When in doubt about the severity of a burn and the need for a referral, consult a burn center. To find a list of burn centers nearest you, go to www.ameriburn.org

Treatment for Burn Injuries

First Degree

- Over-the-counter sprays and gels such as Solarcaine or Aloe will provide moisture and pain relief.
- Self-limiting within a matter of days

Second Degree

- If the patient does not meet criteria for referral to a burn center, determine if the patient or caretaker can provide effective wound care.
- Provide appropriate analgesics as these burns are quite painful especially during dressing changes.
  - Short-term opioids may be necessary.
- Provide initial mechanical debridement of blisters and sloughing epidermis, and then twice daily soap and water washings and thorough drying.
- Appropriate topical agents include:
  - Mupirocin or Polysporin ointment: Apply a small amount with a cotton swab and cover with a secondary nonadherent dressing such as Xeroform, or other petroleum jelly-impregnated gauze, Telfa or Exu-Dry pads followed by a primary dressing such as Kerlix. Recommended twice daily.
    - Silver sulfadiazine (Silvadene) if not allergic to sulfa drugs or products.
- If the patient or caretaker is unable to provide wound care, alternative treatment consists of initial mechanical debridement followed by wrapping the burn in an antimicrobial nanocrystal barrier dressing that can stay in place for up to 7 days. Appropriate products include:
  - Acticoat (Smith & Nephew)
  - Aquacel Ag (Convatec)
  - KerraContact (Crawford)
  - Mepilex Ag (Molnlycke)
  - Promogran Prisma (Systagenix)
  - Tritec Silver (Milliken)

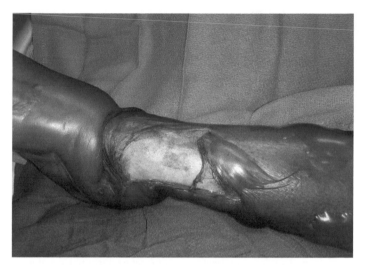

Figure 3.2 Partial/deep partial-thickness burn injury of lower extremity.
Source: Courtesy of Burn and Reconstructive Centers of America.

- Partial-thickness burns generally heal within 2 weeks with weekly follow up recommended. See Figure 3.2
- Many burn centers treat partial-thickness burns of any size with skin substitutes. The healthcare provider should present this to the patient as an option then contact the nearest burn center to transfer care if the patient desires.

Third and Fourth Degree

- These burns always require transfer to a burn center for specialized care. See Figure 3.3.
- Surgical excision and skin substitutes followed by skin grafts are necessary.

Skin Substitutes and Skin Grafts

Skin grafts transplant healthy skin from one part of the body to a well-vascularized wound area. Tables 3.2 and 3.3 define the types of skin grafts.

Cygnus Amnion PatchThis patch is derived from the amnion layer of the placental membrane or umbilical cord.

Amniotic Tissue Allograft

- Cygnus Amnion Patch-derived from the amnion layer of the placental membrane or umbilical cord.
- Epifix/Epiburn-derived from dehydrated human amnion/chorion membrane.

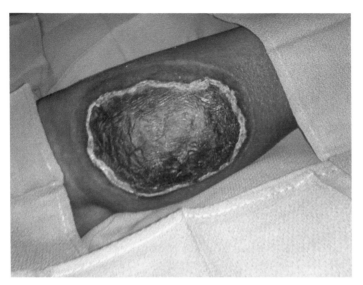

Figure 3.3 Full-thickness burn injury of lower extremity.

Source: Courtesy of Burn and Reconstructive Centers of America.

Table 3.2

Definitions of Skin Grafts

Allograft	Cadaveric grafts, or homograft, transplanted from one individual to another within the same species.
Xenograft	Pig skin grafts, or heterografts, transplanted from an organism of one species to that of a different species.
Autograft	A graft from one part of the body to another part of the same body.

Table 3.3

Graft Types

Split thickness skin graft (STSG)	Contains epidermis and superficial dermis and are often meshed to cover a larger area. Do not have their own blood supply so must be placed on a well-vascularized wound bed.
Full thickness skin graft (FTSG)	Contains epidermis and all the dermis and are used most often to cover smaller defects.

Acellular Allogenic Skin Substitutes

- Integra, Primatrix, Alloderm

Cellular Allogenic Skin Substitutes

- Transyte, Dermagraft, Apligraf

Cultured Epithelial Autografts

Harvesting the patient's own cells to use as a larger epidermal autograft.

Recell

- Spray-On Skin using a small sample of the patient's own skin cells (Avita).

Skin TE

- First-of-its-kind human cellular and tissue-based product derived from a patient's own skin to regenerate full-thickness skin (Polarity).

Bibliography

ABA. (2017). Burn Center Referral Criteria. Retrieved from http://ameri burn.org/wp-content/uploads/2017/05/burncenterreferralcriteria.pdf

Integra Bilayer Matrix Wound Dressing. Retrieved from https://www.inte gralife.com/file/general/1453795598.pdf

Primatrix Dermal Repair Scaffold. Retrieved from www.primatrix.com

Wood, B., Caputy, G., & Kirman, C. (2018, May 10). Skin grafts and biologic skin substitutes. Medscape online. Retrieved from https://emedicine .medscape.com/article/1295109-overview#95

4

Chronic Lower Extremity Wounds

INTRODUCTION

Lower extremity ulcers are the most common chronic wounds, with 80–90% of these wounds being related to chronic venous insufficiency or venous stasis disease. Mixed disease ulcers (both venous and arterial) have been reported in up to 25% of patients with lower extremity ulcers. Studies have shown that at least 25% of patients with diabetes will develop a diabetic foot ulcer and approximately 85% of lower extremity amputations occur due to diabetic foot ulcers.

In this chapter, you will learn:

1. Commonalities and characteristics related to the most common chronic lower extremity wounds, including venous insufficiency ulcers, arterial ulcers, lymphedema, and diabetic ulcers.
2. Indications for established testing procedures to confirm diagnoses.
3. Treatment and therapy priorities.
4. The stages and classification systems for chronic lower extremity wounds.

CHRONIC WOUNDS

Even though it has been said that all chronic wounds start out as acute wounds, always look for a biological or physiological reason why a wound is not healing. Examples of chronic wounds include:

- Pressure injuries
- Diabetic or neuropathic ulcers
- Vascular ulcers
- Wounds secondary to lymphedema

Common characteristics of chronic wounds are:
- Loss of skin and tissue
- Lack of response to conventional types of treatment
- Unapproximated wound edges
- Failure to move beyond the inflammatory phase of wound healing

CHRONIC VENOUS INSUFFICIENCY ULCERS

Venous insufficiency ulcers are classified as either primary or secondary to deep venous thrombosis (DVT). Primary chronic venous insufficiency is the most common and results from valvular incompetence (either reflux or obstruction of venous blood flow) in the superficial veins, deep veins, or perforating veins. The result is venous hypertension of the legs. Early indicators of venous hypertension are leakage around the medial malleolus with skin dyspigmentation, itching, and edema (see Figure 4.1).

Characteristics of Venous Ulcers

- Location: Lower legs and malleolus
- Wound and wound edges: Large and irregular

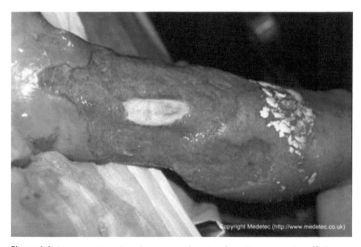

Figure 4.1 Lower extremity ulcer secondary to chronic venous insufficiency.
Source: Metedec.

- Wound bed: Ruddy red with yellow slough
- Exudate: Moderate to large amount
- Appearance of surrounding skin:
  - Macerated, crusted, scaled
  - Hemosiderin staining
  - Pitting edema
  - Hyperpigmentation
  - Lipodermatosclerosis
- Pain level: Dull to severe, cramping in nature, throbbing, not associated with walking or exercise, symptoms improve with leg elevation

Fast Facts

Lipodermatosclerosis: Skin thickening from fibrosis of subcutaneous fat

Testing Procedures

Diagnostic tests help provide a correct diagnosis and identify areas of obstruction, anatomic function, the vascular system involved, and/or other abnormalities contributing to a venous insufficiency ulcer (see Tables 4.1 and 4.2). The results provide the foundation for treatment interventions and therapy.

STAGES OF TREATMENT AND THERAPY PRIORITIES

The selection of treatment and therapy priorities is based on the severity of the disease. Successful treatment is dependent on addressing chronic venous insufficiency with the goals of prevention, management, and treatment of ulcers.

Prevention Stage

The goal is to reduce pooling of blood and to prevent skin breakdown.

- Provide patient education on:
  - Regular exercise and weight reduction
  - Daily skin hygiene (using soap, water, and lotion)
- Elevation of legs above the level of the heart as much as possible
- Begin compression stockings and encourage compliance.

Table 4.1

Diagnostic Testing Procedures for Venous Insufficiency		
Duplex Ultrasonography	Noninvasive	Available with or without color images of the anatomy. B-mode or 2D mode is preferred, as this allows for two-dimensional images.
Trendelenburg test	Noninvasive	Patient's leg is elevated to empty venous blood, the healthcare provider compresses the groin firmly to occlude the greater saphenous vein and the patient stands up, lack of venous filling indicates incompetent valves.
Contrast venography	Invasive	Contrast dye is injected through a catheter in the groin to produce a radiographic picture of the venous system.
Venous photoplethysmography	Noninvasive	Infrared light and a transducer probe are used to assess for venous reflux and muscle pump dysfunction.
Calculation of ankle-brachial index (ABI)	Noninvasive	Calculated by dividing the systolic blood pressure at the ankle by the systolic blood pressure of the arm.

Table 4.2

Ankle-Brachial Pressure Index			
ABPI Value	**Interpretation**	**Action**	**Type of Ulcer, if Present**
> 1.3	Atherosclerosis from PVD	Vascular referral	Venous ulcer
0.95–1.3	Normal range	None	Venous ulcer Compression recommended
0.94–0.80	Acceptable to moderate disease	None	Venous ulcer Can use compression
0.80–0.50	Moderate-to-severe arterial disease	Assess and manage risk factors such as claudication Vascular referral	Mixed ulcers or arterial Light compression only
<0.50	Severe arterial disease	Urgent vascular referral	Arterial; may have gangrene present PVD, peripheral vascular disease.

Management Stage

The goal is to address chronic venous insufficiency by improving venous return.

- Obtain a vascular consult for:
  - Surgical management: Possible vein ligation, phlebectomy, or vein bypass
  - Nonsurgical treatment: Sclerotherapy or endovenous thermal ablation

Treatment Stage

The goal for treating a venous ulcer is to determine what the wound needs.

- Surgical debridement
- Enzymatic debridement
  - Collagenase
  - Medihoney
  - Hydrogel
  - Plurogel
- Provide pain control, infection control, and complex wound care to include debridement
- Choose an appropriate primary dressing based on the amount of exudate and depth of the wound
  - High-to-moderate exudate
    - Aquacel Ag
    - ASSIST Silver
    - Promogran Prisma
  - Low exudate
    - Acticoat
    - KerraContact
    - Mepitel Ag
- Secondary dressing choices
  - Exu-dry
  - Kerlix
- Secure primary and secondary dressings
  - Stretch Net
    - SePro Net
    - Spandage
    - Spandagrip
- Avoid tape that can tear fragile skin
- Use a protectant lotion or barrier on surrounding skin for prevention of maceration

- Discuss the importance of seeing a podiatrist regularly to manage dystrophic toenails
- Educate about the importance of regular follow-up with a wound care specialist

Compression therapy regimens are highly effective in treating chronic venous insufficiency if compliance is maintained.

Compression Therapy

Studies have shown that treating chronic venous insufficiency with compression is key to preventing ulcers and maintaining a healed state. Compression therapy reduces vessel diameter and edema. Higher compression, multilayer systems are more effective than low compression, single-layer bandages. Compression products are divided into categories and vary in action and pressure. Classification is based on the level of compression at the ankle.

- Elastic versus inelastic
- Short versus long stretch
- High compression versus low compression
- Single layer versus multilayer
- Stockings versus bandages versus pumps

Types of Compression Therapy

- Support stockings
  - Static short stretch
  - Custom fit
  - Varying degrees of compression
  - Difficult to apply
  - Example: Jobst
- Orthotic device
  - Static inelastic
  - Must be premeasured
  - Custom fit
  - Easy to apply
  - Example: CircAid
- Zinc Past Bandage
  - Static inelastic
  - Combined dressing and compression in one

- Soothing
- Does not stretch back with pressure changes
- Not a good choice for heavily draining wounds
- Example: Unna Boot
- Four-layer system
  - Static inelastic layers
  - Good choice for heavily draining wounds
  - Adjusts to leg shape
  - Maintains pressure for up to 1 week
  - Examples: Profore, Dynaflex
- Limited-stretch Wraps
  - Static elastic
  - Marks indicate the correct degree of stretch
  - Washable and reusable
  - Examples: Comprilan, Setopress
- Compression pumps
  - Dynamic
  - Safe for patients with arterial disease
  - Can be used at home
  - Require periods of immobility for 2 to 4 hours
  - Usually have to be rented
  - Examples: AV Impulse, Intermittent Pneumatic Compression, Sequential Compression

The common therapeutic compression level is 30-40mmHg at the ankle; however, the healthcare provider may recommend a lower or higher level depending upon the patient's needs.

LYMPHEDEMA

The role of the lymphatic system is to remove toxins, pathogens, and malignant cells. If the lymphatic system is inefficient, fluid accumulates in distal areas, such as the hand or foot, and works its way up the limb as nonpitting edema. Lymphedema is commonly seen after surgery for lymph node dissection and/or radiation therapy for treatment of cancer. It is also associated with accidents or diseases that inhibit proper lymphatic functioning or with infection (see Table 4.3). Eventually, the elasticity of the skin is destroyed, and the skin thickens and becomes severely distorted, a condition known as elephantiasis (see Figure 4.2).

- Primary elephantiasis is inherited as a result of genetic abnormalities.
- Secondary elephantiasis is caused from injury to lymphatic vessels.

Table 4.3

Stages of Lymphedema	
Stage	Description
0	Lymphedema is not present, even though lymphatic vessels have been damaged.
1	Early accumulation of high protein content fluid in the limb; pitting may occur; reversible with rest and elevation.
2	Tissue is spongy and nonpitting; fibrosis is beginning; swelling is not reversible with limb elevation.
3	Severe stage with fibrotic (hard) tissue; swelling is irreversible with affected limb becoming increasingly large.
4	Size and circumference of the limb become noticeably large with skin changes becoming apparent (knobs develop).
5	The affected limb becomes grossly large with deep skinfolds.
6	Knobs cluster together; patient mobility becomes more difficult.
7	The patient may become immobile and handicapped, unable to function independently.

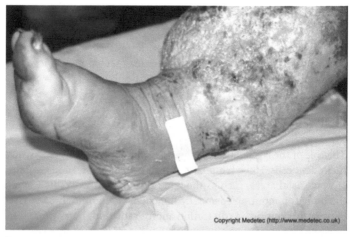

Copyright Medetec (http://www.medetec.co.uk)

Figure 4.2 Lower extremity lymphedema.
Source: Metedec.

Classification of Lymphedema

Grades

- **Grade 1:** Spontaneously reversible with elevation; pitting in nature

- **Grade 2:** Spontaneously irreversible with elevation; nonpitting in nature
- **Grade 3:** Gross increase in limb volume and circumference

Fast Facts

Noninvasive Testing Procedures for Lymphedema

Limb circumference: Use the 2 cm rule: A difference in circumference of 2 cm on either limb is diagnostic.

Stemmer's sign: Gently pinch and lift the skin at the base of the second toe; the test result is positive if the skin cannot be lifted.

Treatment and Therapy

There is no cure for lymphedema, and noncompliance with treatment is common. Treatment can improve quality of life for the patient and is best accomplished by a certified lymphedema therapist. The wound care practitioner can initiate treatment; however, ongoing treatment at a lymphedema center will produce the best outcome for the patient.

Treatment is dependent on establishing the degree of fibrosis and edema. Lymphedema patients require 50 to 60 mmHg of compression as compared to those with venous insufficiency, who require 30 to 40 mmHg. Lymphedema therapy consists of compression, judicious skin care, exercise, weight loss, and manual lymph drainage.

- Manual lymph drainage (MLD)
  - Facilitates contraction of smooth muscles in lymph vessels, which helps to move lymphatic fluid toward the heart
- Intermittent sequential grading pump
  - Helps break up fibrotic hard tissue enabling more efficient lymphatic drainage
- Compression Wrapping
  - Consists of three to four layers of short-stretch bandages that are changed weekly (depending on the amount of exudate)
  - Enhances pump action by providing increased resistance, thereby encouraging lymphatic flow
  - Examples: Profore, Dynaflex, Jobst

Treatment for lower extremity wounds related to lymphedema is similar to chronic venous insufficiency (see Figure 4.3).

Lymphedema Resources
Lymphaticnetwork.org
Lymphnotes.com

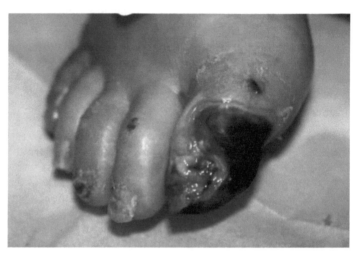

Figure 4.3 Gangrenous toe secondary to arterial insufficiency.
Source: Metedec.

ARTERIAL ULCERS

Arterial ulcers, or ischemic ulcers, are caused by decreased blood flow to the lower extremities, which leads to tissue ischemia.

Characteristics of Arterial Ulcers

- Location: The most distal points, including the toes, ankles, and top of feet (dorsum).
- Wound and wound edges: Small, round, well-defined edges
- Wound bed: Pale, dry base, black eschar is often present
- Volume of exudate: Dry unless the wound is infected
- Appearance of surrounding skin: Shiny with hair loss, thick, dystrophic toenails

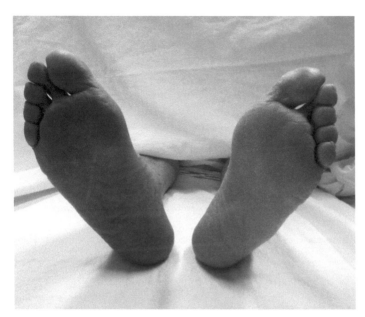

Figure 4.4 Arterial thrombosis causing critical limb ischemia.
Source: Courtesy of Burn and Reconstructive Centers of America.

- Pain level: Very painful; dangling the affected leg will provide some relief

Classifications of Peripheral Arterial Disease (PAD)

The Rutherford-Becker Classification system is useful to categorize the extent and level of PAD and to diagnose Critical Limb Ischemia (see Figure 4.4). Critical Limb Ischemia (CLI) can be diagnosed when the patient has persistent recurring resting pain with non-healing ulceration or gangrene of the foot or toe. See Table 4.4.

- Category 0: Asymptomatic
- Category 1: Mild
- Category 2: Moderate
- Category 3: Severe
- Category 4: Ischemic rest pain
- Category 5: Minor tissue loss such as a nonhealing ulcer or focal gangrene
- Category 6: Major tissue loss above the transmetatarsal level

Table 4.4

Testing Procedures for Arterial Ulcers	
Capillary refill	Normal refill time is less than 3 seconds when the toe pad is pressed.
Skin temperature	Compare one leg to the other and note any difference in temperature.
Ankle-brachial index (ABI)	Compares perfusion pressure of the lower extremity to the upper arm.
Doppler waveforms	Measure the recoil of the artery, loss of elastic recoil of the artery, and occlusion or stenosis.
Lower extremity arterial doppler study	Uses a probe to pinpoint areas of blockage.
Transcutaneous oxygen	Indirect measure of blood flow to the tissue; less than 20 mmHg indicates poor healing potential.

Fast Facts

Any patient with a Rutherford-Becker Category 4 through 6 needs referral to a vascular surgeon.

Indications for Testing Procedures

- Intermittent claudication: Cramping pain and burning in calf muscle that occurs with physical activity but is relieved within 5 minutes of rest
- Nocturnal pain: Cramping pain that occurs when lying down and the leg is elevated
  - Cramping pain that occurs when lying down and the leg is elevated.
- Resting pain: Constant, deep aching pain that is associated with the forefoot, ankle, and toes when the legs are in the dependent position

Guidelines for Obtaining an Ankle-Brachial Index

- Place the patient supine and take their brachial systolic blood pressure in both arms; use the higher systolic reading.
- Place the blood pressure cuff on the affected leg, just above the ankle.

- Place the Doppler probe at a 45-degree angle, at the dorsalis pedis or posterior tibial artery.
- Inflate the cuff until the Doppler signal returns; the point at which you hear the Doppler return is the systolic ankle pressure.
- Divide the ankle pressure by the systolic pressure to obtain the ABI. (Refer to Table 4.3 for ankle-brachial pressure values.)

TREATMENT AND THERAPY PRIORITIES FOR ARTERIAL ULCERS

Prevention

- Educate the patient about the importance of:
  - Smoking cessation (assist with resources)
  - Exercise and weight control
  - Regular follow-up with their primary care provider to ensure control of chronic diseases such as hypertension, hyperlipidemia, chronic renal disease, and diabetes
- Screening
  - The American College of Cardiology and the American Heart Association recommend screening for PAD for anyone over the age of 50 years who has diabetes and/or smokes and anyone over the age of 70 years.

Management Stage

The goal for PAD is to correct the underlying tissue ischemia.

- Obtain a vascular consult for:
  - Surgical intervention: Inflow and outflow procedures such as angioplasty, stents, atherectomy, or bypass
  - Nonsurgical adjunctive treatment: Hyperbaric oxygen therapy or pharmacologic options

Treatment Stage

The goal is to establish a treatment plan for wound care and ultimately heal the ulcer or eliminate the ulcer via amputation, if indicated.

- Control pain.
- Treat infection.
- Determine an appropriate antimicrobial dressing based on the amount of exudate and depth of the wound.

The Six Ps of Critical Limb Ischemia
1. Pulselessness
2. Pain
3. Pallor
4. Poikilothermy (cold)
5. Paresthesia
6. Paralysis

MIXED ARTERIAL AND VENOUS DISEASE

Mixed arterial and venous leg ulcers (MAVLUs) are primarily a result of chronic venous insufficiency and varying degrees of coexisting arterial insufficiency. Studies indicate that approximately 15% of vascular-related lower extremity wounds are of mixed etiology (see Figure 4.5). Management of these complex wounds depends on determining which component is predominant, since compression may not be indicated if considerable arterial disease is present.

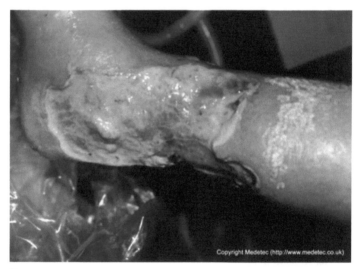

Copyright Medetec (http://www.medetec.co.uk)

Figure 4.5 Lower extremity ulcer secondary to mixed venous and arterial disease.

Source: Metedec.

Characteristics of Mixed Disease Ulcers

- Very painful
- Symptoms of both arterial and venous issues
- ABI between 0.6 and 0.8

Testing Procedures

The following diagnostic tests are used to assist with diagnosing MAVLU.

- Duplex ultrasonography: Arterial and venous
- ABI
- Venography: If deep venous anomaly is suspected
- Arteriography: If revascularization is indicated

Treatment and Management

Treatment of lower extremity wounds secondary to mixed disease mirrors treatment for venous insufficiency and arterial insufficiency. Vascular consultation is necessary to determine the need for invasive and/or surgical intervention. For ABI less than 0.6, revascularization should be the first-line treatment. Patients with ABI values between 0.6 and 0.8 can begin with aggressive wound care, supervised compression, and/or venous ablation. Wounds associated with mixed disease are treated the same as other lower extremity wounds keeping in mind what type of debridement is required and appropriate selection of primary and secondary dressings.

DIABETIC ULCERS

The incidences of diabetes are increasing in staggering numbers. The estimated annual treatment cost of diabetes has risen to $327 billion, an increase of 26% from 2012 to 2017, when the cost was last examined. The American Diabetes Association estimates that more than 34 million Americans have diabetes while an additional 88 million have prediabetes. Diabetic foot ulcerations are one of the most common complications of diabetes, with a worldwide annual incidence of 6.3% (see Figure 4.6).

Diabetes is the single most common cause of all amputations in the United States. Let us stop right here and contemplate amputation. Before there is amputation, there was an ulcer. Before there was an ulcer, there was neuropathy. What if prevention were a paramount? How many lower extremity amputations (LEAs) could be prevented? Studies show that patient education and improved care diminish recidivism with diabetes.

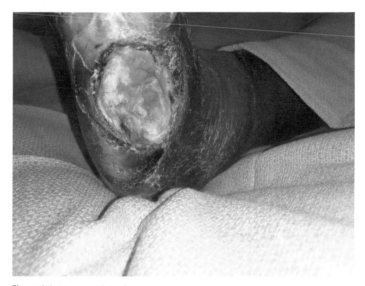

Figure 4.6 Neuropathic ulcer.

Source: Courtesy of Burn and Reconstructive Centers of America.

Diabetic Neuropathy

Nerve disorders caused by diabetes are called neuropathies and are thought to be caused by hyperglycemia and microvascular disease. Nerve damage may be caused, or exacerbated, by other factors such as mechanical injuries, lifestyle factors such as smoking and alcohol use, and autoimmune factors that cause nerve inflammation.

Hyperglycemia Impairs Wound Healing

- Slowing all stages of wound healing
- Blood becomes more viscous, causing abnormal cellular function.
- Higher risk of infection due to impaired host defenses
- Tissue hypoxia results from vascular disease.

Fast Facts

Blood glucose must be controlled to under 200 mg/dL to achieve optimal healing.
Glycosylated hemoglobin (A1c) should be less than 7.
The hemoglobin A1c test shows the average blood glucose over a period of 2 to 3 months.

Types of Neuropathy

Sensory/Peripheral Neuropathy

- Affects arms, legs, feet, and hands
- Symptoms:
  - Paresthesia (tingling, burning, prickling sensations)
  - Insensitivity to pain or temperature
  - Loss of balance, coordination, and deep tendon reflexes

Autonomic Neuropathy

- Affects nerves in the cardiovascular system and internal organs
- Symptoms:
  - Anhidrosis (inability to sweat)
  - Hypoglycemia unawareness
  - Orthostatic hypotension

Motor Neuropathy

- Affects nerves controlling the muscles and can cause muscle atrophy of the feet
- Symptoms:
  - Twitching
  - Muscle cramps
  - Muscle weakness
  - Muscle wasting
  - Foot drop
- History: Alcoholism, obesity, smoking, hypertension, Raynaud's disease, and heredity

Comprehensive Diabetic Foot Exam

- Assess footwear
  - Wide and deep enough to accommodate feet and/or deformities
  - Excessive wear
  - Correct length: There should be a finger length of space between the big toe and end of the insole
  - Socks: Too constricting or worn out
  - Insoles: Worn out or absent
- Foot assessment
  - Xerosis: Rough, dry skin that may have scales or cracks
  - Maceration
  - Blisters
  - Tinea pedis: Fungus
  - Interdigital findings

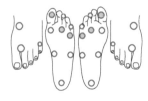

Directions
1. Touch the filament to the skin for 1 to 2 seconds, pushing hard enough to buckle the filament.
2. Place a √ in the circles where the patient feels the filament and an X in circles where sensation is not present.
3. Do not test over calluses, cracks, or the ulcer site.

Figure 4.7 Semmes–Weinstein Monofilament Test.

Source: Courtesy of Health Resources and Services Administration (HRSA), www.hrsa.gov/leap/levelonescreening.htm

- Nail findings
- Calluses
- Preulcerative lesions
- Ulcerations
- Neurological assessment
  - Loss of protective sensation using the Semmes–Weinstein monofilament (see Figure 4.7)
  - Vibratory sensation using a tuning fork on toes and ankles
  - Achilles reflex
- Vascular assessment
  - Pulses: Pedal, dorsalis pedis, posterior tibial, perforating peroneal
  - Color: Rubor or cyanosis
  - Capillary refill time
  - Peripheral edema
  - Temperature comparison between feet
  - ABI and toe-brachial index
- Musculoskeletal assessment
  - Bunions, hammertoes, bone spurs, pes cavus foot type
  - Charcot osteoarthropathy: Midfoot collapse deformity with or without erythema/edema/warmth

Fast Facts

Paperboard-handle monofilaments are affordable and practical. You can order monofilaments at the following sites:
- medicalmonofilament.com
- /www.medline.com

Wagner Classification of Diabetic Foot Ulcers

Diabetic foot ulcers are not staged like pressure injuries. The most common used scale for classifying diabetic ulcers is the Wagner Classification Scale, which grades ulcers based on appearance, depth, and presence of infection. See Table 4.5.

Prevention and Treatment for Diabetic Ulcers

The International Working Group on the Diabetic Foot (IWGDF) has established parameters for risk classification and recommendations for follow-up (see Table 4.6). The goal of treating the diabetic patient is preventing the development of a foot ulcer through:

- Identification of the at-risk foot.
- Regular follow up for foot examinations.

Table 4.5

Wagner Classification Scale	
Grade	Appearance, Location, and Depth of Ulcer
0	Preulcerative lesion, healed ulcers, presence of bony deformity
I	Superficial ulcer without subcutaneous involvement
II	Penetration through the subcutaneous tissue (may have exposed bone tendon, ligament, or joint capsule)
III	Osteitis, abscess, or osteomyelitis
IV	Gangrene of the forefoot
V	Gangrene of the entire foot

Table 4.6

International Working Group on the Diabetic Foot Risk Classification		
Category	Characteristics	Recommended Follow-Up
0	No peripheral neuropathy	Yearly
1	Peripheral neuropathy	Every 6 months
2	Peripheral neuropathy + PAD and/or foot deformity	Every 3–6 months
3	Peripheral neuropathy + history of ulcer or amputation	Every 1–3 months

- Education of patient, care providers, family, and healthcare providers
- Regular wearing of diabetic footwear
- Prompt recognition and treatment of preulcerative wounds
- Wound care is dependent on the Wagner's grading stage but is similar to treatment for pressure injuries.
  - Surgical debridement may be required: Stage IV and V ulcers always need aggressive debridement and often result in amputations at various levels.
  - Enzymatic debridement agents.
  - Choose antimicrobial dressing based on the wound depth and appearance.
  - Offloading is crucial.
- Vascular referral recommended for:
  - All diabetic patients >50 years old.
  - Any patient with decreased or absent pulses or claudication.
- Infectious disease referral recommended for osteomyelitis.
  - Bone culture required.
  - Outpatient antibiotics for up to 6 weeks may be necessary.
- Regular follow-up with footcare specialist for preventative care
- Diabetic education regarding glucose/glycemic control
- Offloading therapy to eliminate abnormal pressure points and prevent ulcer prevention

Fast Facts

Options for the Use of Offloading Therapy
- Total contact casts (the gold standard)
- Removable cast boots (provide better offloading for the forefoot)
- Custom-fabricated ankle–foot orthoses
- Half shoes
- Inlays and insoles (provide least amount of pressure reduction)

Bibliography

American College of Physicians Montana Chapter Meeting (2017, September). The diabetic foot. Retrieved from https://www.acponline.org/system/files/documents/about_acp/chapters/mt/2017/the_diabetic_foot_neibauer.pdf

American Diabetes Association. The staggering costs of diabetes. Retrieved from https://www.diabetes.org/resources/statistics/cost-diabetes

Bell, D. (2012, December). When do you refer a patient for vascular intervention? *Podiatry Today, 25*(12), 1, 3. Retrieved from https://www.woundcare learningnetwork.com

Bell, D. (2020, April). Peripheral arterial disease overview. *Podiatry Management CME*. Retrieved from https://www.podiatry.com

Desai, C. S., Blumenthal, R. S., & Greenland, P. (2014). Screening low-risk individuals for coronary artery disease. *Current Atherosclerosis Reports, 16*(4), 402.

Grada, A. A., & Phillips, T. J. (December 2017). Lymphedema: Diagnostic workup and management. *Journal of the American Academy of Dermatology, 77*(6), 995–1006. http://dx.doi.org/10.1016/j.jaad.2017.03.021

Patel, S., & Surowiec, S. (2020, February). Venous insufficiency. Retrieved from https://www.ncbi.nlm.nih.gov

Perrin, M., Lugli, M., & Malet, O. (2013). Management of mixed arterial and venous lower leg ulcers. *Phlebolymphology, 20*(3), 125–164. Retrieved from https://www.phlebolymphology.org/wp-content/uploads/2014/09/Phlebolymphology79.pdf

Pressure Injuries

INTRODUCTION

Pressure injuries, once known as pressure ulcers, decubitus ulcers, and bed sores, pose significant challenges and burdens to the patient, care providers, and healthcare system in terms of treatment and cost. An average 2.5 million people a year will develop a pressure injury and 60,000 will die because of the complications. It is estimated that between $9.1 and $11.6 billion are spent annually to treat pressure injuries, with $70,000 being spent on a single wound. Pressure injuries are the second most common claim for lawsuits in the United States. This information is very important to healthcare providers, as most pressure injuries have been classified as preventable.

In this chapter, you will learn:

1. The types and stages of pressure injuries.
2. Common tools used to assess pressure injury risk and monitor changes.
3. Measures to prevent the development of pressure injuries.
4. How to treat pressure injuries.

DEFINING PRESSURE INJURIES

Pressure injuries are caused by unrelieved pressure or shear on the skin over bony prominences such as the occiput, scapula, elbow, sacrum, ischium, trochanter, knees, ankles, and heels (see Figure 5.1).

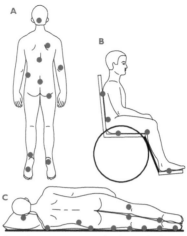

Dots show pressure points when lying on back (A),
when sitting (B), and when lying on side (C).

Figure 5.1 Pressure relief points.

Source: Kifer, Z. (2012). *Fast facts for wound care nursing* (1st ed.). Springer Publishing.

They are characterized by localized damage to the skin or underlying soft tissue.

Risk factors for the development of a pressure injury include:

- Over 65 years of age
- Obesity
- Diabetes
- Cardiovascular disease
- Malnutrition
- Smoking
- Contractures
- Immobility
- Poor skin hygiene
- Restraints
- Spinal cord injuries
- Lying or sitting on hard surfaces
- Residing in a nursing home

Fast Facts

In 2016, the National Pressure Injury Advisory Panel (NPIAP) replaced the terminology "pressure ulcer" with "pressure injury" and changed the use of Roman numerals for staging to Arabic numerals.

STAGES OF PRESSURE INJURIES

Staging pressure injuries is a classification method first designed by Dr. Darrell Shea and modified by the NPIAP. Pressure injury staging is only appropriate for defining the maximum depth of tissue involvement.

Stage 1 Pressure Injury (see Figure 5.2)

- Intact skin with nonblanchable redness
- Darkly pigmented skin may not have visible blanching
- May be painful, firm, and warmer or cooler compared to adjacent tissue.

Stage 2 Pressure Injury (see Figure 5.3)

- Partial-thickness skin loss with exposed dermis
- May appear blistered or abraded
- Wound bed is viable, pink or red, and moist.

Stage 3 Pressure Injury (see Figure 5.4)

- Full-thickness loss of skin with damage to the subcutaneous layers
- Slough and eschar may be present
- Presents as a deep ulcer with or without undermining and tunneling.

Stage 4 Pressure Injury (see Figure 5.5)

- Full-thickness skin and tissue loss with necrosis that may include muscle, bone, or supporting structures such as tendons or joint capsules
- Undermining and sinus tracts are common.

Unstageable Pressure Injury (see Figure 5.6)

- Slough and/or eschar obscures the extent of the damage
- Unable to visualize wound depth.

Deep Tissue Pressure Injury

- Intact or nonintact skin with nonblanchable deep red, maroon, purple discoloration or blood-filled blister
- Discoloration may appear differently on darkly pigmented skin.

Medical Device-Related Pressure Injury

- Results from the use of devices indicated for diagnostic or treatment purposes.
- Stage according to the staging system.

Mucosal Membrane Pressure Injury

- Located on the oral mucosa with a history of medical device use such as an endotracheal tube
- Cannot be staged due to the location.

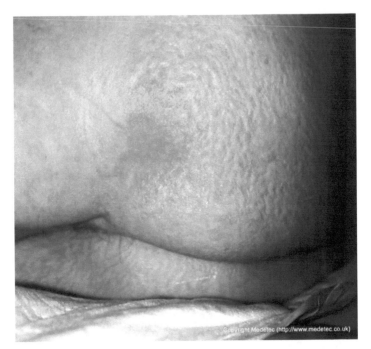

Figure 5.2 Stage 1 pressure injury.
Source: Metedec.

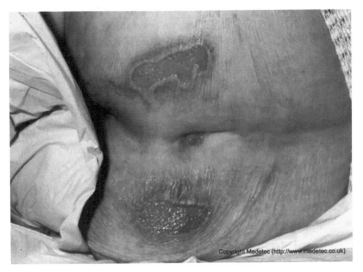

Figure 5.3 Stage 2 pressure injury.
Source: Metedec.

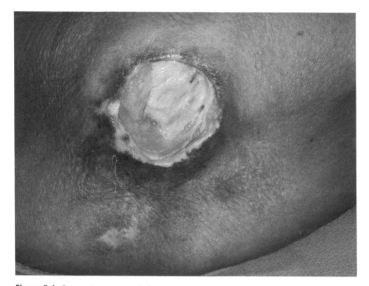

Figure 5.4 Stage 3 pressure injury.
Source: Courtesy of Burn and Reconstructive Centers of America.

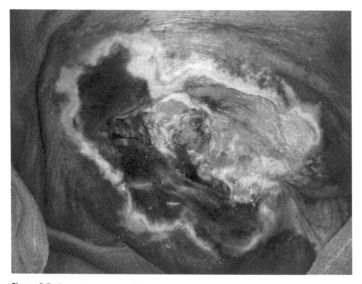

Figure 5.5 Stage 4 pressure injury.
Source: Courtesy of Burn and Reconstructive Centers of America.

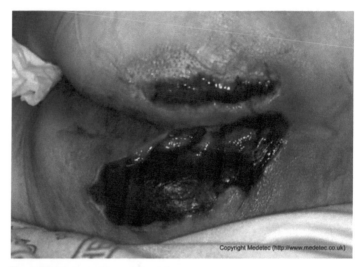

Figure 5.6 Unstageable pressure injury.

Source: Metedec.

TOOLS TO ASSESS PRESSURE INJURIES

The PUSH Tool

The PUSH tool (see Exhibit 5.1) was developed by the NPIAP to monitor changes in pressure injuries. The NPIAP recommends using the tool at least weekly and if the condition of the patient or wound deteriorates. The parameters used by the PUSH tool to score changes are surface area, amount of exudate, and tissue appearance. An increase in the score indicates wound deterioration and necessitates evaluation and possible treatment change.

Other tools used to assess pressure injury status include the Bates-Jensen wound assessment tool and the Sessing Scale. It is more important to provide diligent wound assessment and monitor consistently rather than the specific tool used.

REVERSE STAGING

The NPIAP has issued a position statement regarding reverse staging and recommendations that include the following:

- Never use reverse staging to describe healing pressure injuries related to the anatomical and structural layers of tissue. These tissues are replaced only as scar tissue.
- The maximum anatomic depth, once staged, remains classified at that stage.

- For example, a healing Stage 3 pressure injury or a healed Stage 4 pressure injury.
- Document the progression of healing pressure injuries by characteristics such as size, depth, necrotic tissue, and amount of exudate.
- If a healed pressure injury reopens in the same anatomical site, the wound resumes the previous staging.

Exhibit 5.1.

The PUSH Tool

NATIONAL
PRESSURE
ULCER
ADVISORY
PANEL

Pressure Ulcer Scale for Healing (PUSH)
PUSH Tool 3.0

Patient Name_____ Patient ID# _____

Ulcer Location _____ Date _____

Directions:

Observe and measure the pressure ulcer. Categorize the ulcer with respect to surface area, exudate, and type of wound tissue. Record a sub-score for each of these ulcer characteristics. Add the sub-scores to obtain the total score. A comparison of total scores measured over time provides an indication of the improvement or deterioration in pressure ulcer healing.

LENGTH X WIDTH (in cm²)	0	1	2	3	4	5	Sub-score
	0	< 0.3	0.3 – 0.6	0.7 – 1.0	1.1 – 2.0	2.1 – 3.0	
	6	7	8	9	10		
	3.1 – 4.0	4.1 – 8.0	8.1 – 12.0	12.1 – 24.0	> 24.0		
EXUDATE AMOUNT	0 None	1 Light	2 Moderate	3 Heavy			Sub-score
TISSUE TYPE	0 Closed	1 Epithelial Tissue	2 Granulation Tissue	3 Slough	4 Necrotic Tissue		Sub-score
							TOTAL SCORE

Length x Width: Measure the greatest length (head to toe) and the greatest width (side to side) using a centimeter ruler. Multiply these two measurements (length x width) to obtain an estimate of surface area in square centimeters (cm²). Caveat: Do not guess! Always use a centimeter ruler and always use the same method each time the ulcer is measured.

Exudate Amount: Estimate the amount of exudate (drainage) present after removal of the dressing and before applying any topical agent to the ulcer. Estimate the exudate (drainage) as none, light, moderate, or heavy.

Tissue Type: This refers to the types of tissue that are present in the wound (ulcer) bed. Score as a "4" if there is any necrotic tissue present. Score as a "3" if there is any amount of slough present and necrotic tissue is absent. Score as a "2" if the wound is clean and contains granulation tissue. A superficial wound that is reepithelializing is scored as a "1". When the wound is closed, score as a "0".

- 4 – **Necrotic Tissue (Eschar):** black, brown, or tan tissue that adheres firmly to the wound bed or ulcer edges and may be either firmer or softer than surrounding skin.

- 3 – **Slough:** yellow or white tissue that adheres to the ulcer bed in strings or thick clumps, or is mucinous.

- 2 – **Granulation Tissue:** pink or beefy red tissue with a shiny, moist, granular appearance.

- 1 – **Epithelial Tissue:** for superficial ulcers, new pink or shiny tissue (skin) that grows in from the edges or as islands on the ulcer surface.

- 0 – **Closed/Resurfaced:** the wound is completely covered with epithelium (new skin).

(continued)

Exhibit 5.1 (*continued*)

Pressure Ulcer Healing Chart
To monitor trends in PUSH Scores over time
(Use a separate page for each pressure ulcer)

NATIONAL
PRESSURE
ULCER
ADVISORY
PANEL

Patient Name _____ Patient ID# _____

Ulcer Location _____ Date _____

Directions:
Observe and measure pressure ulcers at regular intervals using the PUSH Tool.
Date and record PUSH Sub-scores and Total Scores on the Pressure Ulcer Healing Record below.

Pressure Ulcer Healing Record											
Date											
Length x Width											
Exudate Amount											
Tissue Type											
PUSH Total Score											

Graph the PUSH Total Scores on the Pressure Ulcer Healing Graph below.

PUSH Total Score	Pressure Ulcer Healing Graph										
17											
16											
15											
14											
13											
12											
11											
10											
9											
8											
7											
6											
5											
4											
3											
2											
1											
Healed = 0											
Date											

www.npuap.org
11F

PUSH Tool Version 3.0: 9/15/98
©National Pressure Ulcer Advisory Panel

Source: From the National Pressure Injury Advisory Panel.

PREDICTING PRESSURE INJURY RISK

If a patient develops a hospital-acquired complication (HAC) such as a pressure injury, it will be tagged with an ICD-9-CM code, meaning that the patient has developed complicating conditions that necessitate increased payments. Because of the Social Security Act 1886(d)

(4)(D) passed in 2005, the increased reimbursement will be denied. The three criteria for designating an HAC were high cost, high volume, and a condition that could reasonably have been prevented through the application of evidence-based guidelines. Therefore, accurate knowledge and strategies for preventing and treating pressure injuries are essential.

Risk assessment forms should be initiated on admission and repeated per facility protocol. Risk assessment tools are used to identify at-risk patients, the level of risk, and the type of risk so that intervention can be started early, when patients are at a mild or moderate level of risk.

The Braden Scale

The most commonly used pressure injury assessment scale is the BradenScale. The Braden Scale stratifies a person's risk for pressure injury development by assessing sensory perception, moisture, activity, mobility, nutrition, and friction (see Exhibit 5.2).

PREVENTING PRESSURE INJURIES

Prioritize preventing a pressure injury from developing when caring for at-risk individuals. Utilize a team approach and include the patient's family and care providers, keeping realistic goals in mind, when managing pressure injuries. Many new dressings, treatment modalities, and pressure injury prevention devices are available to assist wound care providers.

- Eliminate the source of pressure and manage the tissue load (perpendicular force) by addressing the three major factors contributing to pressure injury development: shear, friction, and nutritional debilitation.
  - Turn and reposition at minimum every 2 hours and monitor compliance with documentation and repositioning labels at the foot of the patient's bed.
  - Consider pressure-relieving devices such as low air loss, alternating pressure, air fluidized, or static flotation support surfaces.
  - Offloading footwear, heel protectors, Prevalon boots, positioners
  - Therapeutic linens designed to prevent shear and friction with repositioning
  - Seating cushions: Foam, gel, or air (Roho cushions)

- Limit sitting and head elevation time.
- Use lifting devices and bariatric equipment when needed.
- Manage moisture and incontinence.
- Optimize the environment with infection control practices and nutritional support.
  - Be vigilant with obtaining cultures if the wound is deteriorating or appears infected.

Exhibit 5.2

The Braden Scale for Predicting Pressure Sore Risk

BRADEN SCALE – For Predicting Pressure Sore Risk

| SEVERE RISK: Total score ≤ 9 | HIGH RISK: Total score 10-12 | | DATE OF ASSESS ➡ |
| MODERATE RISK: Total score 13-14 | MILD RISK: Total score 15-18 | | |

RISK FACTOR	SCORE/DESCRIPTION				1	2	3	4
SENSORY PERCEPTION Ability to respond meaningfully to pressure-related discomfort	**1. COMPLETELY LIMITED** – Unresponsive (does not moan, flinch, or grasp) to painful stimuli, due to diminished level of consciousness or sedation. OR limited ability to feel pain over most of body surface.	**2. VERY LIMITED** – Responds only to painful stimuli. Cannot communicate discomfort except by moaning or restlessness, OR has a sensory impairment which limits the ability to feel pain or discomfort over ½ of body.	**3. SLIGHTLY LIMITED** – Responds to verbal commands but cannot always communicate discomfort or need to be turned. OR has some sensory impairment which limits ability to feel pain or discomfort in 1 or 2 extremities.	**4. NO IMPAIRMENT** – Responds to verbal commands. Has no sensory deficit which would limit ability to feel or voice pain or discomfort.				
MOISTURE Degree to which skin is exposed to moisture	**1. CONSTANTLY MOIST** – Skin is kept moist almost constantly by perspiration, urine, etc. Dampness is detected every time patient is moved or turned.	**2. OFTEN MOIST** – Skin is often but not always moist. Linen must be changed at least once a shift.	**3. OCCASIONALLY MOIST** – Skin is occasionally moist, requiring an extra linen change approximately once a day.	**4. RARELY MOIST** – Skin is usually dry; linen only requires changing at routine intervals.				
ACTIVITY Degree of physical activity	**1. BEDFAST** – Confined to bed.	**2. CHAIRFAST** – Ability to walk severely limited or nonexistent. Cannot bear own weight and/or must be assisted into chair or wheelchair.	**3. WALKS OCCASIONALLY** – Walks occasionally during day, but for very short distances, with or without assistance. Spends majority of each shift in bed or chair.	**4. WALKS FREQUENTLY** – Walks outside the room at least twice a day and inside room at least once every 2 hours during waking hours.				
MOBILITY Ability to change and control body position	**1. COMPLETELY IMMOBILE** – Does not make even slight changes in body or extremity position without assistance.	**2. VERY LIMITED** – Makes occasional slight changes in body or extremity position but unable to make frequent or significant changes independently.	**3. SLIGHTLY LIMITED** – Makes frequent though slight changes in body or extremity position independently.	**4. NO LIMITATIONS** – Makes major and frequent changes in position without assistance.				
NUTRITION Usual food intake pattern [1]NPO: Nothing by mouth. [2]IV: Intravenously. [3]TPN: Total parenteral nutrition.	**1. VERY POOR** – Never eats a complete meal. Rarely eats more than 1/3 of any food offered. Eats 2 servings or less of protein (meat or dairy products) per day. Takes fluids poorly. Does not take a liquid dietary supplement. OR is NPO[1] and/or maintained on clear liquids or IV[2] for more than 5 days.	**2. PROBABLY INADEQUATE** – Rarely eats a complete meal and generally eats only about ½ of any food offered. Protein intake includes only 3 servings of meat or dairy products per day. Occasionally will take a dietary supplement OR receives less than optimum amount of liquid diet or tube feeding.	**3. ADEQUATE** – Eats over half of most meals. Eats a total of 4 servings of protein (meat, dairy products) each day. Occasionally refuses a meal, but will usually take a supplement if offered, OR is on a tube feeding or TPN[3] regimen, which probably meets most of nutritional needs.	**4. EXCELLENT** – Eats most of every meal. Never refuses a meal. Usually eats a total of 4 or more servings of meat and dairy products. Occasionally eats between meals. Does not require supplementation.				
FRICTION AND SHEAR	**1. PROBLEM** – Requires moderate to maximum assistance in moving. Complete lifting without sliding against sheets is impossible. Frequently slides down in bed or chair, requiring frequent repositioning with maximum assistance. Spasticity, contractures, or agitation leads to almost constant friction.	**2. POTENTIAL PROBLEM** – Moves feebly or requires minimum assistance. During a move, skin probably slides to some extent against sheets, chair, restraints, or other devices. Maintains relatively good position in chair or bed most of the time but occasionally slides down.	**3. NO APPARENT PROBLEM** – Moves in bed and in chair independently and has sufficient muscle strength to lift up completely during move. Maintains good position in bed or chair at all times.					
TOTAL SCORE	Total score of 12 or less represents HIGH RISK							

ASSESS	DATE	EVALUATOR SIGNATURE/TITLE	ASSESS.	DATE	EVALUATOR SIGNATURE/TITLE
1	/ /		3	/ /	
2	/ /		4	/ /	

| NAME-Last | First | Middle | Attending Physician | Record No. | Room/Bed |

Form 3188P BRIGGS, Des Moines, IA 50306 (800) 347-2345 www.BriggsCorp.com   E304   PRINTED IN U.S.A.
Source: Barbara Braden and Nancy Bergstrom. Copyright, 1988. Reprinted with permission. Permission should be sought to use this tool at www.bradenscale.com
BRADEN SCALE

(continued)

BRADEN SCALE FOR PREDICTING PRESSURE SORE RISK

Patient's Name _____ Evaluator's Name_____ Date of Assessment _____

SENSORY PERCEPTION ability to respond meaningfully to pressure-related discomfort	**1. Completely Limited** Unresponsive (does not moan, flinch, or grasp) to painful stimuli, due to diminished level of consciousness or sedation. OR limited ability to feel pain over most of body.	**2. Very Limited** Responds only to painful stimuli. Cannot communicate discomfort except by moaning or restlessness. OR has a sensory impairment which limits the ability to feel pain or discomfort over ½ of body.	**3. Slightly Limited** Responds to verbal commands, but cannot always communicate discomfort or the need to be turned. OR has some sensory impairment which limits ability to feel pain or discomfort in 1 or 2 extremities.	**4. No Impairment** Responds to verbal commands. Has no sensory deficit which would limit ability to feel or voice pain or discomfort.			
MOISTURE degree to which skin is exposed to moisture	**1. Constantly Moist** Skin is kept moist almost constantly by perspiration, urine, etc. Dampness is detected every time patient is moved or turned.	**2. Very Moist** Skin is often, but not always moist. Linen must be changed at least once a shift.	**3. Occasionally Moist:** Skin is occasionally moist, requiring an extra linen change approximately once a day.	**4. Rarely Moist** Skin is usually dry, linen only requires changing at routine intervals.			
ACTIVITY degree of physical activity	**1. Bedfast** Confined to bed.	**2. Chairfast** Ability to walk severely limited or non-existent. Cannot bear own weight and/or must be assisted into chair or wheelchair.	**3. Walks Occasionally** Walks occasionally during day, but for very short distances, with or without assistance. Spends majority of each shift in bed or chair.	**4. Walks Frequently** Walks outside room at least twice a day and inside room at least once every two hours during waking hours.			
MOBILITY ability to change and control body position	**1. Completely Immobile** Does not make even slight changes in body or extremity position without assistance.	**2. Very Limited** Makes occasional slight changes in body or extremity position but unable to make frequent or significant changes independently.	**3. Slightly Limited** Makes frequent though slight changes in body or extremity position independently.	**4. No Limitation** Makes major and frequent changes in position without assistance.			
NUTRITION usual food intake pattern	**1. Very Poor** Never eats a complete meal. Rarely eats more than ⅓ of any food offered. Eats 2 servings or less of protein (meat or dairy products) per day. Takes fluids poorly. Does not take a liquid dietary supplement. OR is NPO and/or maintained on clear liquids or IVs for more than 5 days.	**2. Probably Inadequate** Rarely eats a complete meal and generally eats only about ½ of any food offered. Protein intake includes only 3 servings of meat or dairy products per day. Occasionally will take a dietary supplement. OR receives less than optimum amount of liquid diet or tube feeding.	**3. Adequate** Eats over half of most meals. Eats a total of 4 servings of protein (meat, dairy products) per day. Occasionally will refuse a meal, but will usually take a supplement when offered. OR is on a tube feeding or TPN regimen which probably meets most of nutritional needs.	**4. Excellent** Eats most of every meal. Never refuses a meal. Usually eats a total of 4 or more servings of meat and dairy products. Occasionally eats between meals. Does not require supplementation.			
FRICTION & SHEAR	**1. Problem** Requires moderate to maximum assistance in moving. Complete lifting without sliding against sheets is impossible. Frequently slides down in bed or chair, requiring frequent repositioning with maximum assistance. Spasticity, contractures or agitation leads to almost constant friction.	**2. Potential Problem** Moves feebly or requires minimum assistance. During a move skin probably slides to some extent against sheets, chair, restraints or other devices. Maintains relatively good position in chair or bed most of the time but occasionally slides down.	**3. No Apparent Problem** Moves in bed and in chair independently and has sufficient muscle strength to lift up completely during move. Maintains good position in bed or chair.				
				Total Score			

- Evaluate and adjust the treatment plan and type of dressing if necessary.
- Be vigilant with utilizing clean procedures with dressing changes and wound care.
- Be attentive to nutritional assessments and laboratory parameters.
- Education is fundamental to quality improvement of pressure injury care and prevention. The NPIAP provides a variety of resources, educational tools, and research information about the many services, tools, experts in the field, and evidence-based practice regarding appropriate intervention for pressure injuries.

TREATING PRESSURE INJURIES

Stage 1 Deep Tissue Injuries and Medical Device-Related Injuries

- Appropriate dressings include:
  - Mepilex
  - Optifoam
  - Allevyn

- Judicious pressure redistribution and/or eliminating the source of injury is priority at this stage to prevent progression.

Stage 2 Pressure Injuries

- Appropriate dressings include:
  - Same products used for Stage 1
  - Mupirocin (Bactroban) or Bacitracin with a nonstick secondary dressing
  - Silver Sulfadiazene Cream (SSD) with secondary dressing such as Exudry
- Judicious pressure redistribution.

Stage 3 Pressure Injuries

- Obtain cultures to identify types of infection and/or colonization and treat with appropriate antibiotics according to culture sensitivities.
- Surgical debridement may be necessary to eliminate necrotic tissue.
- Enzymatic debridement agents
  - Collagenase is most effective.
  - Medihoney
  - Plurogel
  - Hydrogel
- Chemical and mechanical debridement is accomplished by utilizing a wet-to-dry approach utilizing an agent appropriate for the wound and types of organisms identified on culture.
  - Dakin's solution
  - Silver nitrate solution
  - Sulfamylon solution with or without amphotericin B
  - AMD kerlix
- Negative-pressure wound therapy (wound vac)
- Autografts or rotational flaps are an option for closure once infection has been treated and the wound bed is clean and vascularized as evident by returning red granulation tissue.

Stage 4 Pressure Injuries

- Imaging studies to assess for osteomyelitis: Common in the pelvis with chronic pressure injuries.
- Obtain bone biopsy for culture if osteomyelitis is suspected.
- Aggressive surgical debridement is often indicated, including bone.
- Same approach to wound closure as with Stage 3.

- Consult with infectious disease to assist with long-term antibiotics if osteomyelitis is confirmed on bone cultures or if the wound has unusual or resistant organisms.

Unstageable Pressure Injuries

Treatment is dependent on the level of injury that becomes apparent once the skin is no longer intact. Treat initially like Stage 1 injuries and adjust accordingly.

Mucosal Membrane Pressure Injuries

- Remove the source of injury if possible, otherwise, pad and protect the underlying tissue.

Bibliography

Agency for Healthcare Research and Quality. Preventing pressure ulcers in hospitals. Retrieved from www.ahrq.gov

Boyko, T., Longaker, M., & Yang, G. (2018, February). Review of the current management of pressure ulcers. *Advances in Wound Care, 7*(2), 4–8. http://dx.doi.org/10.1089/wound.2016.0697

Industry News. (2016, April 21). National Pressure Ulcer Advisory Panel (NPUAP) announces a change in terminology from pressure ulcer to pressure injury and updates the stages of pressure injury. Retrieved from https://www.woundsource.com/print/blog/national-pressure-ulcer-advisory-panel-npuap-announces-change-in-terminology-pressure-ulcer

The Joint Commission. (2016, July). Preventing pressure injuries. Quick Safety, Issue 25. Retrieved from https://www.jointcommission.org/-/media/deprecated-unorganized/imported-assets/tjc/system-folders/joint-commission-online/quick_safety_issue_25_july_20161pdf.pdf?db=web&hash=A8BF4B1E486A6A67DD5210A2F36E0180

Wound Source Practice Accelerator's Blog. (2018, October 31). Tools of the trade: Pressure injury/ulcer prevention and medical devices. Retrieved from https://www.woundsource.com/print/blog/tools-trade-pressure-injuryulcer-prevention-and-medical-devices

6

Atypical, Complex Wounds

INTRODUCTION

Atypical wounds are difficult acute or chronic wounds that defy normal healing and conservative treatment. These wounds require additional procedures, meticulous surgical debridement or excision, and experienced wound care providers to manage them. Common factors of atypical wounds are conditions such as severe contamination, aggressive infection, and extensive tissue necrosis. Atypical wounds can be confusing, even for wound experts. There is neither universal standardization nor a great deal of evidence-based practice related to such wounds. When addressing atypical wounds, the wound care provider looks for an uncommon etiology as these wounds are not common ulcers related to pressure, diabetes, or venous insufficiency. Atypical wounds are in uncommon locations, have unusual appearances, and react indifferently to common treatment. They can progress rapidly into complex wounds (or possible death) if the underlying cause is not addressed quickly.

In this chapter, you will learn:

1. Initial signs and complications that lead to atypical wounds.
2. How to recognize wounds with extensive tissue necrosis and acute infection.
3. The etiology and characteristics of atypical wounds.
4. The best approach to treatment of atypical wounds.

NECROTIZING FASCIITIS

Necrotizing fasciitis (NF), also known as flesh-eating disease, is a bacterial infection involving skin, soft tissue, and superficial fascia. See Table 6.1. The infection enters the body through a break in the skin caused from trauma, such as a cut or wound, or because of post-surgical complications. Necrotizing fasciitis can occur in any part of the body; however, most often it occurs in the extremities, genitalia, and perineum (Fournier's gangrene). The infection spreads rapidly and can be life-threatening (see Figure 6.1) .

Risk Factors

- Immunosuppression
- Diabetes
- Alcoholism
- Drug abuse

Table 6.1

Types of Soft-Tissue Necrotizing Fasciitis		
Classification	Type of Bacteria	Incidence
Type 1	Gram-positive cocci:	70% to 80%
	Staphylococcus aureus	Most common
	Methicillin-resistant S. aureus	Typically, older patients with multiple comorbidities
	Streptococcus pyogenes	
	Enterococci	
	Gram-negative rods:	
	Escherichia coli	
	Pseudomonas aeruginosa	
	Anaerobes:	
	Bacteroides	
	Clostridium	
Type II	S. pyogenes	20% to 30%
		Mainly affects the extremities
Type III	Vibrio vulnificus	Rare occurrence
		Bacteria found in saltwater
Type IV	Fungal	Rare occurrence
	Candida	Primarily in immunocompromised patients
	Zygomycetes	

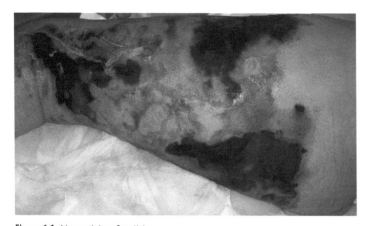

Figure 6.1 Necrotizing fasciitis.

Source: Piotr Smuszkiewicz, Iwona Trojanowska, and Hanna Tomczak.

- Smoking
- Malignancies
- Chronic systemic diseases
- Obesity
- Peripheral artery disease

Signs and Symptoms

Symptoms of NF are usually sudden in onset and escalate rapidly, within a matter of a few days.

- High fever
- Malaise
- Redness and swelling at the site of injury
- Excessive pain
- Rapid progression of redness, swelling, and induration (hardness) beyond the site of injury
- Skin appears shiny and tense
- Skin color progresses from red to purple to black
- Rapid progression to shock

Diagnostic Tests

- Gold standard: Surgical exploration to examine the tissue and fascial plane
- Plain radiography (x-ray)
  - May show subcutaneous gas in the tissue
  - Not sensitive enough to confirm all cases

- CT
  - May show fascial thickening, edema, abscess, or subcutaneous gas
  - More sensitive than plain x-ray
- MRI
  - May show fluid collection within the deep fascia
  - More sensitive than CT
- Elevated white blood cell count (> 15,000 cells/mm^3) and serum sodium <135 mmol/L, elevated serum glucose, elevated C-reactive protein (CRP).

Treatment

- Aggressive surgical excision of infected, necrotic tissue as soon as diagnosis is suspected
  - Multiple surgical procedures are often necessary including procedures for wound closure once all infected tissue has been excised such as:
    - Negative-pressure wound therapy (wound vacs), serial closures, skin grafts
    - Fecal diversion (colostomy) may be necessary for patients with Fournier's gangrene due to the complexity of soft-tissue involvement in the perineum
- Broad-spectrum antibiotics for both Gram-positive and Gram-negative organisms initially
  - Adjust antibiotics to culture sensitivities once obtained.
- Supportive treatment for sepsis
  - IV fluid resuscitation
  - Vasopressors for blood pressure support if necessary
  - Judicious monitoring of urine output
- Pain management
- Hyperbaric oxygen treatments (twice-daily sessions for 20 total)

Prevention

Necrotizing fasciitis can partly be prevented by good hygiene, prompt treatment of wounds (including minor cuts and scratches), and maintaining good glycemic control for diabetes.

VASCULITIS DISORDERS

Approximately 100,000 people in the Unites States are hospitalized every year for vasculitis-related diseases. These disorders (called vasculitides) comprise a group of approximately 20 diseases that involve inflammation of the blood vessels, both arteries and veins. They differ depending on which organs they are associated with, and symptoms range from mild to life-threatening. Vasculitis is classified as either large vessel, medium vessel, or small vessel depending on the size of the affected vessel. See Table 6.2. Vasculitis is considered an autoimmune disorder primarily caused by leukocyte migration. These conditions can take years to be diagnosed due to the varying presentations and symptoms. Complications of vasculitis include stroke, heart attack, gangrene, gastrointestinal perforations, and renal failure.

Signs and Symptoms

- Fever, malaise, weight loss
- Purpura: Widespread violaceous skin lesions that can lead to ulcerations and necrosis
- Muscle pain and inflammation, joint pain, and swelling
- Neuritis, headache, tinnitus, visual loss
- Hypertension
- Nose bleeds, hemoptysis, lung infiltrates
- Abdominal pain, bloody stool

Diagnostic Tests

- Biopsy of the involved organ or tissue
- Angiography to assess for patterns of inflammation in the vessels
- 18F-fluorodeoxyglucose positron emission tomography/computed tomography (FDG-PET/CT) to assess for enhanced glucose metabolism in affected vessels

Table 6.2

Major Type of Vasculitis	
Vasculitis	**Affected Organs**
Cutaneous small vessel	Skin, kidneys
Granulomatosis with polyangiitis	Nose, lungs, kidneys
Eosinophilic with polyangiitis	Lungs, kidneys, heart, skin
Behcet's disease	Sinuses, brain, eyes, skin, lungs, kidneys, joints
Kawasaki disease	Skin, heart, mouth, eyes
Buerger's disease	Hands and feet
Takayasu's arteritis	Aorta and lower extremity vessels
Wegener's granulomatosis	Systemic effect on multiple organs. See Figure 6.2.

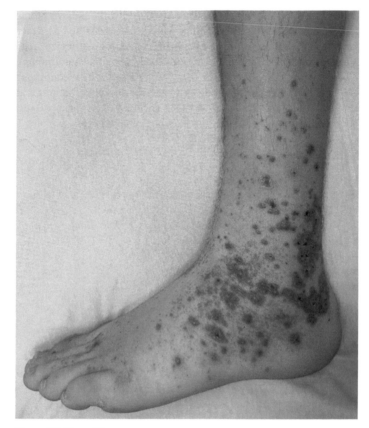

Figure 6.2 Vasculitis.

Source: Dr. James Heilman.

- Laboratory tests that indicate inflammation
  - Increased erythrocyte sedimentation rate (ESR)
  - Increased C-reactive protein (CRP)
  - Anemia
  - Increased white blood cell count
  - Eosinophilia
  - Elevated antineutrophil cytoplasmic antibody (ANCA)
  - Hematuria
- Other organ function tests may be abnormal.

Treatment

The goal of treatment for vasculitis is to stop the inflammatory response, suppress the immune system, and help affected organs improve function.

- Corticosteroids such as prednisone
- Immune suppression agents such as cyclophosphamide
- Antibiotics if infection is suspected
- Conservative wound care if necessary; elevation and compression of the affected extremity
  - Debridement of necrotic tissue: surgical, enzymatic, chemical, or mechanical
  - Wound cultures
    - Antibiotics according to culture sensitivities
  - Maintain moist wound environment to promote cell migration
  - Select dressing according to amount of wound exudate

Fast Facts

The gold standard for helping establish a definitive diagnosis for complex or atypical wounds is tissue biopsy of the affected tissue or organ.

CALCIPHYLAXIS

Calciphylaxis is a metabolic disorder associated primarily with renal failure and has an annual mortality of 40% to 80%. The etiology occurs from occluded blood vessels by vascular calcifications that result in necrotic wounds that are difficult to heal. Uremic calciphylaxis develops in end-stage renal disease while nonuremic calciphylaxis occurs in patients with some renal function (see Figure 6.3).

Risk Factors

- Renal failure: Dialysis or renal transplant patients
- Hyperphosphatemia
- Hypercalcemia
- Hyperparathyroidism and hypoparathyroidism
- Vitamin K deficiency
- Warfarin use
- Obesity
- Diabetes
- Female sex

Signs and Symptoms

- Severe pain often disproportionate to the skin findings
- Reticulated (net-like) violaceous skin discoloration
- Confluent, indurated (hard) plaques

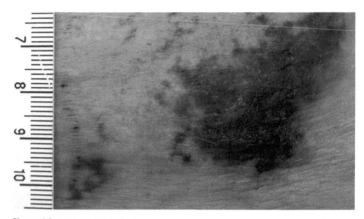

Figure 6.3 Early calciphylaxis.

Source: Courtesy of Niels Olson.

- Skin nodules
- Progression to deep, necrotic ulcers
- Superinfection of wounds and cellulitis

Diagnostic Tests

- Tissue biopsy/punch biopsy taken from the margin of the lesion (preferably two specimens) from different sites
  - Histology will confirm vessel or dermal calcifications
- Bone scan
- Laboratory tests to include:
  - Calcium
  - Phosphorus
  - Alkaline phosphatase
  - Parathyroid hormone
  - Vitamin D
  - Liver function tests
  - Renal function tests (Blood, Urea, Nitrogen [BUN], creatinine)

Treatment and Prevention

Aggressive surgical management is not indicated for wounds associated with calciphylaxis. If the wounds are grossly necrotic or infected, initial surgical debridement may be indicated. The goal for treatment in calciphylaxis is to stop vascular calcifications.

- Dialysis
- Elimination of triggers such as warfarin, corticosteroids, iron
- Modifying doses of calcium and vitamin D supplements

- Sodium thiosulfate during dialysis
- Sensipar to control parathyroid hormone
- Parathyroidectomy
- Pain management
- Hyperbaric oxygen therapy can benefit recalcitrant wounds.

Wound care measures should focus on mechanical or chemical debridement and appropriate topical agents to help minimize bacterial colonization and provide an optimal environment for healing with dressings that focus on moisture control. Appropriate wound care agents include:

- Collagenase, Medihoney, hydrogel, Plurogel
- Sodium hypochlorite (Dakin's solution)
- AMD kerlix
- Puracyn
- Silver nitrate solution
- Silver sulfadiazine cream (SSD)

PYODERMA GANGRENOSUM

Pyoderma gangrenosum is a rare inflammatory skin disorder that begins as papules or nodules that eventually become painful ulcerations. If not recognized and treated promptly, the ulcerations spread and worsen. See Table 6.3.

The exact cause is unknown, although it is classified as an autoimmune disorder. Approximately 50% of people with pyoderma gangrenosum have an underlying systemic inflammatory bowel condition such as Crohn's disease or ulcerative colitis, while approximately 25% of patients have arthritis (most often rheumatoid). Malignancies, such as leukemia, are the most common disease associated with pyoderma gangrenosum (see Figure 6.4).

Signs and Symptoms

- Small, red bumps or blisters
- Painful erosive ulcerations
- Well-defined violaceous-colored border to wounds
- Pustules
- Chronic fungal skin infections
- Secondary symptoms related to the underlying causative disorder

Diagnostic Tests

No specific tests exist to diagnose pyoderma gangrenosum. Tissue biopsy generally shows no specific features, but rather, it assists to establish

Table 6.3

The Four Variants of Pyoderma Gangrenosum

Type	Location	Characteristics
Classic	Most commonly seen on legs but can occur on any skin surface; can occur near surgical stomas (peristomal)	Small pustules that enlarge and spread rapidly; violaceous border; undermined ulcer edge
Pustular	Trunk, arms, legs	Groups of pustules that coalesce and form a large ulceration; usually persist for months; most often associated with inflammatory bowel disease
Atypical or bullous	Arms, hands, and face	Superficial blisters that spread rapidly; more superficial ulcers; violaceous, undermined wound edge; most often associated with hematological malignancies
Vegetative	Can occur on any skin surface	Chronic lesions; painless; usually occurs as a single lesion; responds more readily to treatment

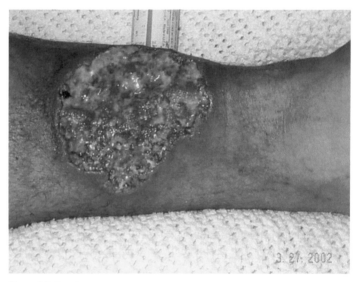

Figure 6.4 Pyoderma gangrenosum.
Source: Courtesy of Chronie.

differential diagnoses that can be contributing to the skin manifestations. Diagnosing pyoderma gangrenosum is based on patient history, clinical assessment and findings, and exclusion of other conditions.

Treatment

- Immunosuppression is the mainstay of treatment
  - Corticosteroids
  - Cyclosporine
  - Cyclophosphamide
  - Tacrolimus
  - IV immune globulin
- Topical anti-inflammatory, antibacterial creams and ointments
  - Corticosteroids
  - Dapsone
- Conservative wound care until the underlying cause is identified and treated.
  - Dakin's solution
  - Puracyn
  - Enzymatic debriding agents if needed
  - Collagenase
  - Medihoney
- Skin grafts once the inflammation is controlled

Fast Facts

Many complex, atypical wounds are the manifestation of an underlying disease process; therefore, identifying the cause is key to understanding what is driving the wound when establishing a treatment plan.

HIDRADENITIS SUPPURATIVA

Hidradenitis suppurativa (acne inversa) is a chronic, progressive, autoinflammatory disorder that affects the apocrine glands in warm, moist, hair-bearing areas such as the axillae, groin, mons pubis, perineum, and breast folds. Less commonly, the scalp and face can also be affected. The lesions associated with hidradenitis progress to abscesses with sinus tracts and cause significant scarring. Hidradenitis is the most severe condition in dermatology and causes significant psychological impact to the affected person in terms of impaired body image, depression, anxiety, sexuality, and ability to be self-sufficient. See Table 6.4.

Hidradenitis most often starts in puberty and is most active in young adulthood (see Figure 6.5). Prevalence of hidradenitis is inaccurate but is thought to vary between 1% and 4% of the population.

Risk Factors

- Female sex
  - Three times more common in women and often resolves at menopause
- Family history of hidradenitis
- Obesity
- Cigarette smoking
- Follicular disorders such as acne conglobata and pilonidal cysts
- Inflammatory bowel disease
- Acne
- Psoriasis
- Hirsutism

Diagnosis

The diagnosis of hidradenitis suppurativa is based on the patient's medical history and physical assessment findings. Often misdiagnosed, it can take years for a patient to get an accurate diagnosis, as most healthcare providers are not familiar with the disease. Cultures can be taken from sites of abscesses to assist with appropriate antibiotics. Histology generally identifies acute and chronic inflammation with abscess formation; however, it is important to rule out malignancy with this disease.

Table 6.4

Hurley Staging for Hidradenitis Suppurativa	
Stage	Characteristics
Stage 1 (mild)	Single or multiple abscess formation; no sinus tract or scar formation at the site of healing wounds
Stage II (moderate)	Single or multiple recurrent abscesses with tract formation and scar formation at the site of healing wounds; widely separated lesions
Stage III (severe)	Diffuse involvement of multiple, interconnected abscesses and tracts

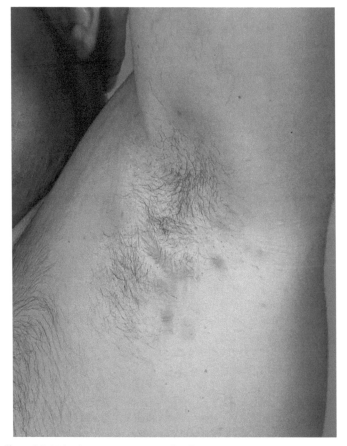

Figure 6.5 Hidradenitis suppurativa of axilla.

Source: Courtesy of Ziyad Alharbi, Jens Kauczok, and Norbert Pallua.

Treatment

Successful treatment for hidradenitis requires a multidisciplinary approach from both a medical and surgical standpoint and should include expert wound care specialists, dermatology, infectious disease, psychiatry, and surgeons. Patients must be educated that treatment is lengthy and difficult. Medical management involves:

- Weight loss
- Smoking cessation
- Good hygiene with antibacterial soaps
- Pain control
- Mental health referral for depression, anxiety, social isolation

- Topical clindamycin
- Topical benzoyl peroxide
- Prolonged courses of antibiotics to control inflammation
- Combination antibiotic therapy for severe disease
  - Clindamycin or doxycycline with rifampin for 6 to 12 weeks
- Antiandrogen therapy
  - Oral contraceptives
  - Spironolactone
  - Finasteride
- Immunotherapy
  - Intralesional corticosteroids
  - Systemic corticosteroids
  - Methotrexate or cyclosporine
  - Biologic agents such as adalimumab

Surgical management for hidradenitis suppurativa involves:

- Incision and drainage of acute abscesses
- Wide excision of areas with diffusely involved, persistent lesions with subsequent skin grafting of the area
- Laser ablation
- Temporary fecal diversion with colostomy if the perianal area is involved.

Fast Facts

Patients and healthcare providers can find more information and resources about hidradenitis suppurativa at: www.hs-foundation.org

BROWN RECLUSE AND BLACK WIDOW SPIDER BITES

Spider bites are an external cause of an atypical wound. Brown recluse spider bites are generally painless, while a black widow bite causes acute pain within minutes.

Signs and Symptoms

- Tremors
- Muscle cramps
- Dizziness
- Chest pain

A brown recluse spider bite causes development of a necrotic wound at the site usually 2 to 4 hours after the bite. Fang marks may be present with a deep-purple plaque around the center and a clear halo with redness at the bite periphery. This is called "the red, white, and blue sign." Venom from both spiders is neurotoxic.

Treatment

- Broad spectrum antibiotics for cellulitis
- Elevation if the affected area is an extremity
- Surgical or mechanical debridement if the necrosis is extensive or causing cellulitis
- Wound care depending on the depth and involvement of the wound
  - Wet to dry with Dakin's solution or Puracyn
  - Bactroban or SSD
  - Enzymatic debridement if needed
    - Collagenase
    - Thera-honey
    - Plurogel or hydrogel

STEVENS-JOHNSON SYNDROME AND TOXIC EPIDERMAL NECROLYSIS SYNDROME

Stevens-Johnson syndrome (SJS) and toxic epidermal necrolysis syndrome (TENS) are serious skin conditions of acute onset that occur as a reaction to certain medications or infections and can be life-threatening. Both conditions affect the epidermal layer of the skin, mucous membranes, and the soft-tissue layer that lines the digestive tract from mouth to anus. Other affected areas are the eyes and reproductive organs.

Mortality is directly associated with total body surface area skin involvement and slough and is as high as 50%. SJS causes epidermal sloughing of less than 10% total body surface, while TENS reactions cause epidermal sloughing of greater than 30% total body surface area (see Figure 6.6). An intermediate combination diagnosis is given when 10% to 30% is involved.

Most cases of SJS and TENS are caused by an allergic reaction to medications. There are many drugs known to have a greater propensity to trigger SJS/TENS and include:

- Sulfa drugs (trimethoprim sulfamethoxazole/Bactrim)
- Anti-epileptic drugs
- Allopurinol
- NSAIDs
- Antibiotics

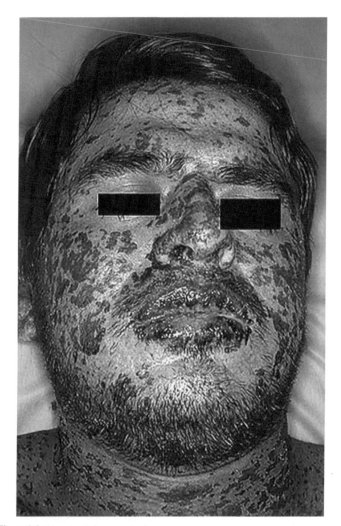

Figure 6.6 Stevens-Johnson syndrome.

Source: Courtesy of Dr. Thomas Habif.

Symptoms

SJS and TENS are often misdiagnosed. Obtain a thorough history on patients presenting with a combination of these symptoms combined with risk factors and act early to begin treatment.

- Skin pain is a common symptom.
- High fever > 100.4°F

- Headache
- Body aches
- Joint pain
- Cough
- Rash that quickly develops into blisters and skin sloughing
- Facial swelling
- Conjunctivitis
- Lip peeling and crusting
- Painful urination

Diagnosis

SJS and toxic epidermal necrolysis syndrome are easily diagnosed by tissue biopsy and patient presentation based on amount of skin sloughing. A positive Nikolsky's sign is a helpful diagnostic aid.

Fast Facts

Nikolsky sign: A skin finding in which the top layer of skin (epidermis) can be separated from the middle layer (dermis) by rubbing with the thumb.

Treatment

- IV immunoglobulin 1 gm/kg/day for 72 hours should be initiated immediately on diagnosis.
- H1 and H2 blockers
  - Pepcid + Benadryl or Allegra + Benadryl
- Proton pump inhibitor (PPI)
  - Protonix
- Replacement fluids with lactated Ringers
- Oral hygiene including mouthwash that contains anesthetic agents
  - Magic mouthwash
  - Buccal swabs and prevention of gingival adhesions
- Eyedrops or ointments
  - Artificial tears
  - Tobradex ointment
  - Ophthalmology consult is recommended.
- Nutritional support
  - Enteral feeds via feeding tube may be necessary for patients with severe oral mucosa involvement and large surface area slough.
- Multimodality regimen for pain management

- Vaginal care to prevent vulvovaginal sequelae
  - Betadine douches
  - Intravaginal glucocorticoid ointments
  - Vaginal molds for significant involvement (adults only)
- Broad-spectrum antibiotics
- Skin care for <10% TBSA
  - AMD kerlix
  - Aquacel Ag
  - Xeroform for face/vaginal areas/gluteal cleft
- Surgical debridement for large surface area involvement with placement of skin substitute
  - Amnion (Permaderm)
  - Allograft
  - Xenograft
  - Nanocrystaline silver dressing over skin substitute
    - Acticoat
    - Exsalt
    - Assist Silver
- Resolving SJS/TENS
  - Bactroban/Bacitracin/xeroform to open areas
  - Beta GlucanPro to healed areas
  - Compression/scar management

Treatment for SJS and TENS is like that of burn patients in that a large surface area of skin is involved. Complications such as dehydration, severe infection, and sepsis can develop within days if not recognized and treated promptly. Patients with these conditions are best managed at a burn center, and prompt transfer should be arranged.

KENNEDY TERMINAL ULCER

The Kennedy terminal ulcer (KTU) is irreversible, unavoidable skin breakdown that occurs in some people who are dying. First documented by Dr. Jean Martin Charcot in 1877 (the same physician who researched and described Charcot foot), this phenomenon was later redocumented by Karen Lou Kennedy and the staff at Byron Health Center in Fort Wayne, Indiana, in 1989.

The ulcer develops within days in people who are terminally ill and is not considered a pressure injury. The exact etiology of KTUs is unclear; however, clinicians believe they are likely a cause of the organs and body functions failing.

Characteristics of a KTU are as follows:

- Location: Sacrococcygeal area primarily but can be elsewhere such as the buttocks

- Appearance: Irregular edges, asymmetrical shape
- Dark, bruised color that progresses rapidly to an ulcer
- Not treatable
- Treatment focuses on palliative care.

Bibliography

Alharbi, Z., Kauczok, J., & Pallua, N. (2012, June). A review of wide surgical excision of hidradenitis suppurativa. *BMC Dermatology, 12*(9). Retrieved from https://bmcdermatol.biomedcentral.com/articles/10.1186/1471-5945-12-9

Brooklyn, T., Dunnill, G., & Probert, C. (2006, July). Diagnosis and treatment of pyoderma gangrenosum. *BMJ, 333*(7560) 181–184. Retrieved from https://www.ncbi.nlm.nih.gov/pmc/articles/PMC1513476/

Calciphylaxis. Retrieved from https://www.mayoclinic.org/diseases-conditions/calciphylaxis/diagnosis-treatment/drc-20370562

Chang, J. (2019, May). Calciphylaxis: Diagnosis, pathogenesis, and treatment. *Advances in Skin and Wound Care, 32*(5), 205–215. Retrieved from https://nursing.ceconnection.com/ovidfiles/00129334-201905000-00003.pdf

Cleveland Clinic. Stevens-Johnson syndrome. Retrieved from https://my.clevelandclinic.org/health/diseases/17656-stevens-johnson-syndrome#:~:text=Stevens-Johnson%20Syndrome%20(SJS),with%20this%20condition%20are

Duong, T. A., Valeyrie-Allanore, L., Wolkenstein, P., & Chosidow, O. (2017). Severe cutaneous adverse reactions to drugs. *Lancet, 390*(10106): 1996–2011. http://dx.doi.org/10.1016/S0140-6736(16)30378-6. PMID 28476287. S2CID 9506967

Habif, T. Stevens-Johnson Syndrome. Retrieved from http://www.dermnet.com/images/Stevens-Johnson-Syndrome

Holland, K. (2018, June 15). Kennedy ulcers: What they mean and how to cope. Updated March 7, 2019. Retrieved from https://www.healthline.com/health/kennedy-ulcer

Lebwohl, M. Pyoderma gangrenosum. Retrieved from https://rarediseases.org/rare-diseases/pyoderma-gangrenosum/

Maffioli, L., & Mazzone, A. (2014). Giant-cell arteritis and polymyalgia rheumatica. *NEJM, 371*(17), 1652–1653. http://dx.doi.org/10.1056/NEJMc1409206. PMC 4277693. PMID 25337761

McMillan, K. (2014, June). Hidradenitis suppurativa: Number of diagnosed patients, demographic characteristics, and treatment patterns in the United States. *American Journal of Epidemiology, 179*(12), 1–3. Retrieved from https://pubmed.ncbi.nlm.nih.gov/24812161/

NHS. Stevens-Johnson syndrome. Retrieved from https://www.nhs.uk/conditions/stevens-johnson-syndrome/#:~:text=Stevens%2DJohnson%20syndrome%20is%20usually,eventually%20dies%20and%20peels%20off

Schank, J. (2018, February). The Kennedy terminal ulcer—alive and well. *Journal of the American College of Clinical Wound Specialists, 8*(1–3), 54–55. http://dx.doi.org/ 10.1016/j.jccw.2018.02.002

Shanmugam, V., Angra, D., Rahimi, H., & McNish, S. (2017, March). Vasculitic and autoimmune wounds. *Journal of Vascular Surgery: Venous and*

Lymphatic Disorders, 5(2), 280–292. Retrieved from https://www.ncbi
.nlm.nih.gov/pmc/articles/PMC5319730/

Smuszkiewicz, P., Trojanowski, I., & Tomczak, H. (2008). Late diagnosed
necrotizing fasciitis as cause of multiorgan dysfunction syndrome: A
case study. *Cases Journal, 1*(125) Retrieved from https://casesjournal
.biomedcentral.com/articles/10.1186/1757-1626-1-125

II

Assessment, Measurement, and Documentation

7

Assessing Wounds

INTRODUCTION

All assessment is perpetual work in progress.

-Linda Suske

Do not allow making assessments intimidating. Think about wound assessment in terms of the analogy that just because you've seen one human face doesn't mean that you've seen them all, or that you will ever see them all. However, as Vince Lombardi said, "Practice does not make perfect. Only perfect practice makes perfect." Continually assessing wounds will improve your skills and make you more effective in developing your treatment plans. Take time with your assessments and really scrutinize what you are seeing.

In this chapter, you will learn:

1. The components that comprise an accurate wound assessment.
2. How to obtain a patient history, as this will be the first indicator of the patient's intrinsic ability to heal.
3. How to assess various aspects of pain by asking the patient questions about their pain and by using a pain scale.
4. How to manage pain by minimizing aggravating factors or providing analgesia.

COMPONENTS OF WOUND ASSESSMENT

An accurate wound assessment is the first step in a wound care plan. The assessment provides baseline data and records ongoing changes, which measures the effectiveness of the treatment plan, and interventions related to the progression of the wound's status. The mnemonic ASSESSMENT helps make sure that all elements of wound assessment are covered.

Fast Facts

ASSESSMENT
A- Anatomic location of wound
S- Size, shape, and stage
S- Sinus tract, tunneling, undermining, fistula
E- Exudate
S- Sepsis (systemic or local)
S- Surrounding skin
M- Maceration
E- Edges, epithelialization
N- Necrotic tissue
T- Tissue bed

Anatomic Location

- Specify the wound location on the patient's body.
- Keep in mind that more than one wound may be present.

Determine the Wound Etiology

- Venous ulcer
- Arterial ulcer
- Mixed ulcer
- Diabetic (neurogenic) ulcer
- Pressure injury

Size, Shape, and Stage

- Include wound measurements in centimeters width, length, and depth
- Oval, round, irregular, butterfly
- Stages 1 to 4 or deep tissue injury or unstageable for pressure injuries
- Wagner's stage for diabetic ulcers

Sinus Tract, Tunneling, Undermining, Fistula

- Sinus tract: infection drainage pathways from deep tissue or bone to an opening on the skin surface
- Tunneling: Passageway underneath the skin that can extend in any direction through soft tissue; it results in dead space and the threat of abscess formation
- Undermining: Tissue destruction that extends under and along the wound edges
- Fistula: An abnormal connection between an organ, vessel, or intestine and another structure
- Document the extent and location using the clock face position with 12 o'clock being the patient's head and 6 o'clock being the feet
- Document using centimeters

Exudate

- Type of exudate (drainage)
  - Serous (clear, thin, watery plasma)
  - Serosanguineous (yellow, pink tinged)
  - Sanguineous (bloody and thick)
  - Purulent (pus)
- Amount of exudate
  - Minimal
  - Light
  - Moderate
  - Heavy

Sepsis Indicates Wound Appears Infected

- Systemic
- Local
- Both
- Wound malodor

Surrounding Skin

- Assess the wound's periphery
  - Erythema (redness)
  - Edema (swelling)
  - Intact
  - Indurated (hard)
  - Temperature
  - Color
  - Moisture
  - Dry, cracked

Maceration

- Location if present

Edges, Epithelialization

- Attached or not attached
- Rolled under (epibole): This requires removal of the rolled-under edges that can be achieved by scrubbing the edges until they bleed, applying silver nitrate sticks to the edges, and surgical excision
- Fibrotic, scarred
- Surgical incision approximated or not
- Sutures/staples present
- Epithelialization present or not

Necrotic Tissue

- Yellow slough
- Eschar (soft or hard)
- Soft or stringy
- Percentage of wound involved

Tissue Bed

- Red granulation present or not
- Hypergranulation
- Moist or dry
- Pain or tenderness

OBTAINING A PATIENT'S HISTORY

An expert wound care practitioner does not just simply slap a dressing on a wound. Instead, the practitioner establishes the patient's expected wound outcome. The goal for wound care and healing should be realistic and established early. The patient's history is the first indicator of their intrinsic ability to heal.

There are three main components of a patient's wound care history:

1. The patient's overall health and well-being, including:
   a. Nutrition
   b. Psychological history
   c. Cultural history
   d. Causative factors
   e. Chronic diseases
   f. Compliancy

g. Care setting
h. Economic status
i. Medications
j. Home life or homelessness
k. Occupation
l. Smoking status
m. Substance use
2. The head-to-toe physical assessment and review of systems
3. The wound history

Fast Facts

Questions to ask in obtaining a wound history:
- When did you first notice the wound? Is this the first time you have had it?
- Does it hurt? (Use pain scale.)
- Has it changed in size, odor, or appearance?
- Who takes care of the wound?
- What have you been putting on the wound?

There are two easy, but important, tests to be done during an initial assessment for any patient with diabetes and/or with a lower extremity wound: one for arterial perfusion of the lower legs and the other for protective sensation of the feet.

1. Ankle-brachial index (ABI): A simple comparison of perfusion pressures in the lower legs with those in the upper arms (refer to Chapter 4).
2. Semmes-Weinstein monofilament examination: A simple test to determine sensation in the feet (refer to Chapter 4).

Recognizing Pain

Pain is inevitable. Suffering is optional.

-Anonymous

If you were to excel in only one type of assessment, it should be accurate and continuous pain assessment. It is our responsibility as clinicians to identify and treat pain. As Margo McCaffery, MS, RN-BC, FAAN, said, "A patient's pain is what they say it is" plain and simple, and should never be neglected. The American Pain Society identifies pain as "the fifth vital sign."

Asking the patient the following questions will help you to assess their pain:

1. Where is the pain?
2. Does it radiate?
3. When did the pain start and is it ongoing?
4. Is the pain aching, burning, cramping, deep, sensitive, stinging, and so on?
5. What causes the pain, that is, dressing changes, debridement, infection, position changes?

Pain Scales

- FACES pain rating scale: Good to use with children (see https://wongbakerfaces.org/wp-content/uploads/2016/05/FACES_English_Blue_w-instructions.pdf).
- Numeric rating scale (NRS): Commonly considered the gold standard, this is an 11-point Likert-type scale where zero means no pain and ten means worst possible pain (see Exhibit 7.1).

Fast Facts

An absence of facial expression or response when performing a seemingly painful procedure does not mean that the patient is free of pain.

Managing Pain

The goal of pain management is to identify the cause of pain, eliminate the source of pain, and/or provide analgesia. As described in Table 7.1, WHO developed a three-step analgesic ladder, progressing from nonopioids to opioids (with or without adjuvants) as needed to achieve an adequate and acceptable level of pain relief for the patient. The WHO ladder is a good guideline for mild to severe pain. The WHO pain ladder's key principles are:

- By the clock
  - Drugs should be given routinely around the clock rather than on an as-needed basis.
- By mouth
  - The oral route is the preferred route of administration
  - If the oral route is not feasible, the least invasive route should be used.

Exhibit 7.1

Numeric Rating Scale

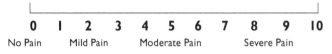

Numeric Rating Scale (NRS)

| 0 | 1 | 2 | 3 | 4 | 5 | 6 | 7 | 8 | 9 | 10 |

No Pain   Mild Pain   Moderate Pain   Severe Pain

Source: D'Arcy, Y. (2011). *Compact clinical guide to chronic pain management*. New York: Springer Publishing.

Table 7.1

The WHO Pain Relief Ladder

Reported Pain Level	Class of Medication to Use	Adjuvant Medication
Step one: 1 to 3 (mild pain)	Nonopioid analgesics: NSAIDs or acetaminophen	With or without an adjuvant
Step two: 4 to 6 (moderate pain)	Weak opioids: Hydrocodone, codeine, tramadol	With or without an adjuvant
Step three: 7 to 10 (severe pain)	Strong opioids: Morphine, methadone, fentanyl, oxycodone, buprenorphine, tapentadol, hydromorphone, oxymorphone	With or without adjuvant

- By the ladder
  - Administration of drugs should follow the order outlined in the pain relief ladder.

Adjuvant medications are used to treat side- effects and provide additional analgesia. The clinician should re-evaluate adjuvants every time analgesics are changed. Examples include:

- Antidiarrheal agents
- Antidepressants
- Antipsychotics
- Laxatives
- Antiemetics

- Anticonvulsants
- Topical anesthetics
- Topical steroids

WHO guidelines state that, "Relief of psychological, social, and spiritual problems is paramount. Attempting to relieve pain without addressing the patient's non-physical concerns is likely to lead to frustration and failure."

Bibliography

Anekar, A., & Cascella, M. (2020, January). WHO analgesic ladder. NCBI Bookshelf. Retrieved from https://www.ncbi.nlm.nih.gov/books/NBK554435/

Ayello, E. A. (2004, November–December). Elements of wound assessment. *Advances in Skin and Wound Care, 17*(9), 461.

F314 Federal Regulations of Pressure Sores: 12 Components of Wound Assessment and Documentation. ARKANSAS INNOVATIVE PERFORMANCE PROGRAM (AIPP). Skin Management Tool Kit. Retrieved from https://www.google.com/search?q=12+components+of+wound+assessment+and+documentation &oq=12&aqs=chrome.1.69i57j012i46j69i6013.141140j4&sourceid=chrome&ic=UTF-8#

8

Documenting and Photographing Wounds

INTRODUCTION

"If you didn't document it, it didn't happen."

-Anonymous

A wound care practitioner's documentation should provide information about thorough assessments, interventions, and patient's responses to wound care treatment. The wound care practitioner should document accurate and complete wound evaluations, treatment modifications, and outcomes. Documentation serves as the primary communication tool among all members of the healthcare team. Thorough documentation provides legal defense, verifies communication, and provides rationales for treatment decisions and modifications. Documentation and photographs provide evidence of wound progress or failure. Moreover, healthcare facilities get reimbursed based on accurate wound documentation.

In this chapter, you will learn:

1. Why accurate wound documentation is so important.
2. How wound documentation affects reimbursement.
3. Requirements for wound documentation.
4. The importance of photographing wounds and techniques.

IMPORTANCE OF WOUND DOCUMENTATION

Clear and concise wound documentation demonstrates patients are receiving appropriate care, communicates the patient's plan of care to other members of the team, and captures the appropriate complexity of the patient's condition. These data have implications on billing and coding, as failure to capture reportable diagnosis and procedures directly affects reimbursement from the Centers for Medicare and Medicaid Services (CMS) and other health insurance companies. Inpatient hospital facilities who bill Medicare Part A for reimbursement use the International Classification of Diseases, 10th Revision, Clinical Modification (ICD-10-CM) to report both diagnoses and billable medical interventions or procedures such as wound debridement. Outpatient settings use ICD-10-CM to report diagnoses and Current Procedural Terminology (CPT) codes to report medical interventions. Consequently, the documentation for capturing accurate diagnosis codes is similar for both inpatient and outpatient settings, while documentation to support wound care treatment varies.

The Office of the Inspector General (OIG) of the U.S. Department of Health and Human Services states "Providers carry the burden of proving that care was actually rendered to patients (residents). If healthcare providers are unable to prove that they rendered appropriate care because it was not documented, the OIG and other fraud enforcement agencies may conclude that claims submitted are false." The Social Security Act mandated "the establishment of minimum health and safety standards that must be met by providers and suppliers participating in the Medicare and Medicaid programs." CMS provides regulatory guidance to healthcare providers through the State Operations Manual (SOM). Appendix PP of the SOM contains minimum standards for wound care documentation with emphasis on long-term care facilities.

These standards are specifically found in Section 483.25 of Appendix PP of the SOM, which includes F-tags. F-tag 686 (Treatment/Services to Prevent/Heal Pressure Injuries) specifically addresses minimum assessment, monitoring, and documentation requirements as related to pressure injuries. F-684 addresses requirements for any wound. Facilities that fail to meet these specific mandates can receive an F-tag, which results in decreased reimbursement and poor-quality scores.

To help ensure compliance regarding necessary care, healthcare facilities should make sure wound documentation meets or exceeds the requirements set forth in F-686. Facilities should have a system that ensures daily monitoring with periodic documentation of measurements (minimum weekly) and consistent terminology and documentation.

Documentation Requirements

Many standardized assessment tools exist for documenting wound care; however, many healthcare facilities now utilize Electronic Medical Records (EMRs). Wound EMRs have greatly improved wound data collection through use of templates that allow clinicians to enter individualized wound assessments and the plan of care accurately and efficiently. Most wound EMRs can capture digital images of wounds as well.

Both paper forms and EMRs should address the components of wound assessment discussed in Chapter 7. Accurate wound documentation should include:

1. Visual inspection
   a. Anatomic location (See Table 8.1).
   b. Size (length x width x depth)
   c. Existence of sinus tract, undermining, tunneling
   d. Shape
   e. Exudate
   f. Condition of surrounding skin
   g. Edges
   h. Appearance of the wound bed

Table 8.1

Terminology for Documenting Anatomic Locations		
Location	Term	Definition
Hands	Palmar	Toward the palm
	Dorsal	Top of the hand
Feet	Plantar	Bottom of feet
	Dorsal	Top of feet
Body	Medial	Toward the middle
	Dorsal	Relating to the back or posterior of a structure
	Posterior	The back or underside
	Anterior	The front
	Superior	Above or toward the top
	Inferior	Below or toward the bottom
	Lateral	Toward the side

2. Stage of wound
   a. Stage of pressure injury and/or type
   b. Pressure injury risk assessment (Braden scale)
   c. Wagner's stage (diabetic ulcers)
3. Changes in wound condition
4. Wound category changes (e.g., deep tissue injury evolves to a Stage 4 pressure injury)
5. Patient responses/behaviors
   a. Pain level
   b. Refusal of care/treatment
   c. Overall patient condition
6. End-of-life wounds
   a. Distinguish Kennedy terminal ulcers from other pressure injuries or wounds
7. Health Insurance Portability and Accountability Act (HIPAA)-appropriate wound photos
8. Unavoidable pressure injuries
   a. Document risk factors, comorbidities, conditions
9. Document all calls to a physician or other clinician such as a nurse practitioner or physician assistant
   a. Include orders received and your response
   b. Treatment modifications
10. Patient or family education
11. Nutritional status
    a. Most EMRs can automatically incorporate lab values and body mass index (BMI)
12. Treatments/procedures
    a. Include instruments used for sharp debridement
    b. Include supplies used for wound care
13. Referrals given or recommended
    a. Nutrition
    b. Podiatry
    c. Vascular
    d. Infectious disease

IMPORTANCE OF WOUND PHOTOGRAPHY

Digital wound photography provides objective, consistent wound assessment and can readily track trends in wound healing.

Digital wound images:

- Facilitate forming accurate diagnosis.
- Enhance clinical documentation.
- Help monitor wound progress.

- Help prevent wound litigation.
- Allow communication among providers.
- Create staff accountability.

The American Professional Wound Care Association has established guidelines for the use of digital images and photographing wounds. The guidelines are:

- Use the same camera for all photographs.
  - Same image resolution.
  - Same angle, source of light, and intensity.
  - Same lens magnification for digital cameras.
- Maintain the camera's distance, rotation, angle, and height from the wound.
  - Make sure the wound is in the same position in all images.
  - All images in a sequence should be either predebridement or postdebridement.
- Use patient stickers to identify the patient.

Photographing of patients' wounds falls under the HIPAA of 1996 which states that the patient must provide informed consent to be photographed. If photographing of wounds will be routine, informed consent can be written into the facilities admission documents. If the digital images will be used for a manuscript or presentation, the patient or legal representative must be informed and provide additional written consent.

Fast Facts

Digital Wound Software
- RxPhoto
- eKare
- Healthy.io
- 3D Wound Management
- Silhouette
- SWIFT skin and wound
- HealthEpix
- Wound Matrix.

Bibliography

Centers for Medicare and Medicaid Services. Long-Term Care Facility Resident Assessment Instrument 3.0 User's Manual. Version 1.15. Released October 2017.

Ericson, C. (2014 Journal). Successful documentation of wound care. *Wound Care Advisor, 3*(3). Retrieved from https://woundcareadvisor.com/successful-documentation-of-wound-care-vol3-no3/

Krasner, D. (2018, January 25). Wound documentation do's and don'ts: 10 Tips for success. Woundsource blog. Retrieved from https://www.woundsource.com/blog/wound-Documentation-dos-donts-10-tips-success

Office of Inspector General Website. Retrieved from https://oig.hhs.gov/fraud/strike-force/

State Operations Manual Appendix PP-Guidance to Surveyors for Long Term Care Facilities. Revised November 22, 2017. pp. 248–266, 272, 273.

Three reasons digital wound photography is key to better skin outcomes. Retrieved from https://www.medline.com/skin-health/digital-wound-photography/

III

Wound Care Treatment and Protocols

9

Selecting the Correct Dressings

INTRODUCTION

Wound care dressings can be complex. Work to stay abreast of manufacturers and the latest technology in wound care offerings. Get to know your wound care product representatives. They can offer you invaluable education about their products. Ask to see a sample, open and feel it, and compare others in the same category.

Dressings can be divided into two categories: primary and secondary. Primary dressings make contact with the wound bed and often contain antimicrobial agents. Secondary dressings secure primary dressings in place. Sometimes, they are both the same. Wound care specialists need to be competent in understanding the products by category, their application techniques, and how cost-effective they are. Can (and should you) use one product with another? How often do you change a particular dressing? Knowing the answers to these questions is a good example of wound care competency. This chapter will help you become more competent with your wound care choices.

In this chapter, you will learn:

1. Components of the ideal wound dressing.
2. The various categories of wound products and dressings and their indications for use.
3. The advantages and disadvantages of the different wound care products and dressings.

FUNCTIONS OF THE IDEAL WOUND DRESSING

There are well over 6,000 wound care products available for use today. Textile-based dressings are being manufactured from a variety of different materials and can be considered "smart dressings." An ideal wound dressing should address the following properties:

- Creates an optimal moist environment at the wound bed.
- Protects the wound from secondary infection.
- Allows for gaseous exchange.
- Eliminates and/or absorbs exudate.
- Provides mechanical protection.
- Decreases necrotic tissue from the wound.
- Is comfortable and adaptable.
- Is able to be removed without causing trauma to the wound and excess pain.
- Is cost-effective.

Other considerations when deciding which dressing to choose are:

- Is the wound partial or full thickness?
- What will the wound be cleaned with?
  - Use noncytotoxic wound cleanser.
  - Consistent use of wound cleansing products.
- Does the wound have tunneling or undermining?
  - Will it have to be packed?
- How often will the dressing need to be changed?
  - Less exudate allows for longer wear times.
  - Wounds heal faster when the wound bed is kept covered with a consistent temperature.
- Is the dressing going to conform to the type and location of the wound?
  - The dressing should be easy to apply and remove.
  - The dressing should be comfortable and adhere to the specific anatomical location of the wound.
- How much is the wound draining? (See Exhibit 9.1.)
  - Dressings should appropriately absorb the amount of assessed exudate.
  - Larger size dressings will protect the periwound from maceration with high exudate wounds.
- What size dressing will the wound require?
- Who will be changing the dressing?
  - The patient or caregiver must be able to demonstrate competency with dressing changes.

Exhibit 9.1

Selecting Dressings According to Amount of Exudate

Amount of Exudate			
None	Low	Moderate	High
	Gauze		
Films			
Hydrogel			
	Hydrocolloid		
		Alginate	
		Foam	
			Superabsorbent

- ▪ Always select a dressing that does not need to be changed every day if the wound condition allows.
- ■ Who is the payor source?
  - ▪ Most payors have a specific list of reimbursable products.
  - ▪ Some insurance companies require preauthorization if other products need to be used.

Fast Facts

Wounds are either digressing, unchanging, or progressing. Choose the primary dressing based on whether the wound is dirty or clean, wet or dry, and deep or shallow. Choose the secondary dressing based on minimal or heavy drainage and the condition of the surrounding skin.

Dressing Reapplication

Dressing reapplication is based on physician orders, product insert recommendations, and facility guidelines. Compare these and use good judgment. If the primary dressing indicates a daily change and you choose a secondary dressing that indicates a 3-day change, you will change the dressing according to the shortest reapplication time. Make sure that your dressing selections are safe, appropriate, and cost-effective.

WOUND DRESSING CATEGORIES

Alginates

Definition

- Nonwoven fibers derived from sterilized brown seaweed or kelp.

Indications

- Heavily draining wounds/ulcers
- Chronic venous insufficiency
- Surgical wounds
- Cavities/craters

Advantages

- Highly absorptive
- Protect wound from infections
- Easy to apply
- Can be used under compression
- Reapplication time is 1 to 3 days depending on the type of wound and amount of exudate

Disadvantages

- Require a secondary dressing
- Not indicated for bleeding or dry wounds
- Not used for wounds with minimal exudate

Products

Algicell by Derma Sciences

Algisite by Smith & Nephew

Aquacel by Convatec

Caclcicare by Hollister

Curasorb by Covidien

Kaltostat by Convatec

Maxorb II or extra by Medline

Medihoney by Derma Sciences

Melgisorb by Molnlcyke

Nu-Derm by Systagenix

Reliamed by ReliaMed

Safe n simple by Simplicity

Silverlon by Argentum

Silvercel by Systagenix

Sorbalgon by Hartmann

Tegaderm high gelling and high integrity by 3M

Antimicrobial Topical Dressings

Definition

- Contain ingredients capable of inhibiting or destroying microorganisms

Indications

- For use on infected wounds or to prevent infections
- For use on skin tears or traumatic wounds
- To cover and protect skin grafts and donor sites

Advantages

- Available in a variety of forms
- Can control bioburden
- Broad-spectrum coverage
- Many can stay intact for up to 7 days

Disadvantages

- Can cause hypersensitivity
- Can require a secondary dressing
- Frequency of change varies according to product

Products

Acticoat by Smith & Nephew	Iodoflex by Smith & Nephew
Assist Silver by Milliken	Kerra Contact by Crawford
Exsalt by Crawford	Mepilex AG by Molnlycke
Hydrofera Blue by Healthpoint	Mepitel AG by Molnyycke

Collagens

Definition

- Contain collagens derived from bovine, equine, porcine, or avian sources
- Aid fibroblast production
- Contribute to new tissue growth

Indications

- Pressure injuries
- Venous ulcers
- Donor sites
- Vascular wounds
- Diabetic ulcers
- Surgical wounds
- Traumatic wounds

Advantages

- Some products interact with exudate to form a gel
- Available in a variety of forms
- Can be used with antimicrobials

- Flexible and comfortable
- Controls bioburden

Disadvantages

- Require a secondary dressing
- Not indicated for necrotic wounds
- May need to be changed twice daily on a wound with heavy exudate

Products

Biopad by L&R USA

Biostep by Smith & Nephew

Colactive Plus by Covalon

Collatek Collagen Gel by Human BioSciences

Cutimed Epiona by Essity

Dermacol by DermaRite

Endoform Natural by Aroa Biosurgery Ltd

Fibracol by 3M+KCI

Gentell Collagen by Gentell

Helix3 by Amerx HealthCare Crop

Hycol by Sanara Med tech

Hyprochon by Hymed

Mckesson Collagen by McKesson

Medifill II by Human BioSciences

Promogran by 3M+KCI; Puracol by Medline

Simpurity by Safe n Simple

Skin Temp by Human BioSciences

Stimulen by Southwest Technologies

Triple Helix by MPM Medical

Foams

Definition

- Highly absorptive polyurethane or polymer dressings that wick exudate away from the wound bed

Indications

- Apropriate for any wound
- Match product to amount of exudate

Advantages

- Available with or without borders
- Different sizes, shapes, and thicknesses
- Can be impregnated with antimicrobials or enzymatic debridement agents

- Easy to apply and remove
- Reapplication time is 3 to 5 days

Disadvantages

- May cause maceration to surrounding skin if not changed appropriately
- Not indicated for wounds with eschar

Products

Abena by Abena

Allevyn by Smith & Nephew

Cardinal Health Silicone by Cardinal

Coloplast Biatain by Coloplast

Convatec by Convatec

Derma Xtrasorb by Dumex Derma Sciences

Dermarite by DermaRite

Hollister Triact by Hollister

Hydrofera Blue by Appulse Medical

Gemcare 360 by Gemcare

Kendall Copa Island by Covidian+Medtronic

Mepilex by Molnlycke

MPM by MPM

Optifoam by Medline

Reliamed Foam by Reliamed

Restore by Hollister

Simplicity by Safe n Simple

Systagenix Tielle Plus by Systagenix+Acelity

Tegaderm by 3M

Zemifoam by Zemi Medical

Hydrocolloids

Definition

- Wafer-style dressings derived from gelatin, pectin, polysaccharides, or sodium carbomethylcellulose
- Turns into a gelatinous covering

Indications

- Primary or secondary dressing for minimally draining wounds
- Preventive dressing on nonfragile skin

Advantages

- Occlusive in nature (the most adhesive dressing available)
- Can be impregnated with antimicrobials

- Assist with autolytic debridement
- Available in a variety of sizes, shapes, forms
- Reapplication time is 3 to 7 days

Disadvantages

- Not recommended for wounds with heavy exudate
- Can be difficult to remove
- Can emit odor with removal

Products

Abena Hydrocolloid by Abena

Cardinal Thin by Cardinal

Coloplast Trial by Coloplast

Comfec Plus by Coloplast

Covidian Ultec Pro Alginate by Covidian

Conco Flexicol by Covalon

Cutimed Hydro L by BSN Medical

Duoderm by Convatec

Exuderm by Medline

Gemcare 360 Hydrocolloid by GemCare 360

Hartmann Flexicol by Hartmann USA

Mckesson Hydrocolloid by McKesson

Reliance Hydrocolloid by Reliance

Restore by Hollister

Tegaderm Hydrocolloid by 3M.

Hydrogel

Definition

- Water or glycerin based.

Indications

- Painful wounds
- Skin tears
- Dry wounds
- Minor burns

Advantages

- Available in a variety of forms and sizes
- Very flexible
- Soothing and hydrating

Disadvantages

- Require a secondary dressing
- Not recommended for heavily draining wounds

Products

Amerigel by Amerx	Excel-Gel by MPM
Aquaflo Hydrogel by Covidien	Intrasite Gel by Smith & Nephew
Aquasite by DermaSciences	Normlgel by Molnlycke
Curafil/Curagel by Covidien	Regenecare Hydrogel by MPM
Cutimed Gel by BSN Medical	Reliamed Hydrogel by ReliaMed
Derma-Gel by Medline	
Dermagran by Derma Sciences	Restore by Hollister
	Skintegrity by Medline
Deroyal Mutlidex by DeRoyal	Solosite Hydrogel by Smith & Nephew
Duoderm Gel by ConvaTec	Tegaderm Hydrogel by 3M
Elasto-Gel by Southwest	

Composites

Definition

- Multiple layers that combine distinct components into a single product to provide multiple functions

Indications

- Indicated for a variety of wounds

Advantages

- Act as bacterial barrier, absorption, and adhesion
- Available in an assortment of sizes, shapes, and products
- Can function as a primary or secondary dressing
- Can be used with topical medications

Disadvantages

- Not indicated for Stage 4 pressure injuries
- Adhesive border can limit use on fragile skin
- Not all provide a moist wound environment

Products

3M Medipore by 3M+KCI

3M Tegaderm by 3M+KCI

Alldress Absorbent by Molnlycke

Cardinal Composite by Cardinal

Covaderm Plus by DeRoyal

Covrsite PLS by Smith & Nephew

Dermadress by DermaRite

Drysee by Drysee

Dupress by Integra Life Sciences

Dynaguard by Dynarex

Genteel Comfort by Genteel

Hydrofilm Plus by Hartmann

Mckesson Barrier Island by McKesson

Mepore PRO by Molnlycke

Mpm Multi-Layer by MPM

Opsite by Smith & Nephew

Repel by MPM

Stratasorb by Medline

Suresite 123 by Medline

Telfa Plus by Cardinal.

Contact Layers

Definition

- Woven or perforated, nonadherent products placed on a wound or graft site for protection

Indications

- Primary dressing for partial or full-thickness wounds with minimal to heavy exudate, infected wounds, donor sites, skin graft sites
- Can be used with topical medications

Advantages

- Conform to shape of the wound
- Porous, protective
- Come in a variety of sizes
- Do not need to be changed with every dressing change

Disadvantages

- Not indicated for Stage 1 pressure injuries, full-thickness burns, tunneling wounds, shallow wounds, dry wounds, or eschar
- Require a secondary dressing

Products

3M Tegaderm by 3M

Adaptic by 3M+KCI

Atrauman by Hartmann

Colactive by Covalon

Conformant by Smith & Nephew

Covrsite by Smith & Nephew

Dermanet by De Royal

Drynet by Smith & Nephew

Kerra Contact + AG by 3M+KCI

Mckesson Contact by McKesson

Mepitel One and Mepilex by Molnlycke

Multipad by De Royal

N-Terface by Winfield

Profore by Smith & Nephew

Rylon-1 by Biomed

Silicone Contact by Cardinal

Silverlon by Argentum Medical

Telfa Clear by Cardinal

Tritec by Milliken

Urgotul by Urgo Medical

Gauze

Definition

■ Woven or nonwoven, adherent or nonadherent, sterile or unsterile rolls, pads, strips, or sponges

Indications

■ Variety of wounds for absorption, packing, primary or secondary dressing

Advantages

■ Available in a variety of sizes, shapes, and forms
■ Promote a moist wound environment
■ Provide protection and mechanical debridement
■ Can be impregnated with antimicrobial agents

Disadvantages

■ May adhere to fragile skin, wounds, or skin grafts
■ Can cause maceration if not changed appropriately
■ Dry out easily

Products

ABD Pads by Medline

Abdominal PADS by ReliaMed

Amd Kerlix by Cardinal

Cosmopore by Hartmann

Drawtex by Drawtex

Duform by Derma Sciences

Exu-Dry by Smith & Nephew

Gauze Sponges by Dukal

Curity Iodoform, Excilon, Conform, Kerlix Rolls, and Telfa by Covidien

Packing Strips by Medline

Pak-Its by Integra Life Sciences

Woundgard by MPM.

Super Absorbent

Definition

- Multilayer products of highly absorptive fibers, such as cellulose, cotton, rayon, or polymers that lock fluid in the dressing and converts it to a gel

Indications

- Wounds that are highly draining and wet such as with chronic venous insufficiency

Advantages

- Minimize maceration of periwound
- Require fewer dressing changes
- Outer layer provides pressure redistribution and cushioning
- Available in many sizes and shapes

Disadvantages

- Not indicated for wounds that are bleeding or tunneling
- Some are not compatible with solutions
- Not recommended for dry wounds

Products

Covawound by Covalon

Cutimed by Essity

Eclypse by Advancis Medical

Devrasorb by Curaline

Xtrasorb by Integra Life Sciences

Flivasorb by L&R USA

McKesson Super by Mc Kesson.

Petrolatum and Oil Emulsions

Definition

- Sterile gauze dressing impregnated with an oil emulsion blend

Indications

- Donor sites
- Graft sites
- Low-to-moderate draining wounds

Advantages

- Nonadherent and nonadhesive
- Promote moist wound environment
- Allow exudate to flow onto secondary dressing

Disadvantages

- Not indicated for heavily draining wounds
- May cause hypersensitivity or allergic-type reaction

Products

Cardinal Xeroform

Dermarite Xeroform

Dynarex Oil Emulsion Dressing

Genteel Xeroform

Petrolatum Impregnated Gauze

Simplicity Xeroform

Vaseline Petrolatum Gauze

Dressing Retention

Definition

- Elastic and tubular stretch dressings
- Cut to size and shape
- Secure dressings in place while allowing ease of movement and air circulation

Indications

- For patients with tape sensitivities, difficult areas to dress, restless patients

Advantages

- Easily removed for dressing changes
- Reusable

- Inexpensive
- Does not cause trauma to the wound or surrounding skin

Disadvantages

- Application learning curve for using the right size

Products

Elastic Net by Medline

Flexinet and Surgilast by Derma Science

Medigrip by Medline

MT Spandage by Medi-Tech

Stretch Net by DeRoyal

SE Pro Net by Medical Action Industries

Systenet Premium by Integra Life Sciences

Tubigrip and Tubifast by Molnlycke.

Films

Definition

- Clear film dressings made from polyurethane- added polymers allow for gaseous exchange and moisture to escape

Indications

- Minimally draining wounds with nonfragile surrounding skin

Advantages

- Fewer dressing changes, reduce friction, available in a variety of shapes and sizes
- Transparent to allow wound assessment

Disadvantages

- Can adhere to fragile skin
- Can cause maceration
- Can cause trauma to skin if not removed properly

Products

Bioclusive by Systagenix

Comfeel by Coloplast

Gemcare 360 by Gemcare 360

Hydrofilm by Hartmann

Mckesson Transparent by McKesson

Mepore by Molnlycke

Opsite by Smith & Nephew

Reliamed by ReliaMed

Skin-Prep Protective by Smith & Nephew

Suresite by Medline

Tegaderm by 3M.

Scar Therapy

Definition

■ Products that help reduce the appearance of scars

Indications

■ For patients with hypertrophic or keloid scars

Advantages

■ Reduce texture and elevation of scars

Disadvantages

■ Not all scars respond to these products

Products

Cica-Care by Smith & Nephew

Jobskin Garments by Torbot Group

Medigel Z by Medical Z

Mepiform by Molnlycke

Oleeva Clear Silicone by BioMed Sciences.

Wound Closures

Definition

■ Products that help approximate the edges of a wound

Indications

■ For gaping wounds and wounds left open to heal by tertiary intention

Advantages

■ Variety of sizes, shapes, and forms
■ Some absorb into the skin

Disadvantage

■ May damage fragile skin
■ Application learning curve
■ May require tension/pressure to apply or after application

Products

Abra Surgical by Acell

Dermabond by Ethicon

Dermaclose by Wound Care Technologies

Episeal by De Royal

Indermil by Connexicon Medical

Leukostrip by Smith & Nephew

Medi-Strips by Medline

Montgomery Straps by Medline

Octylbond by Sourcemark

Stay-Strips by DermaRite

Steri-Strip by 3M+KCI

Suture Strip and Shur-Strip by Integra Life Sciences.

NEGATIVE-PRESSURE WOUND THERAPY

Negative-pressure wound therapy (NPWT), also known as vacuum-assisted wound closure (wound vac), is a system that applies subatmospheric pressure, either continuously or intermittently, to a wound. This negative pressure encourages vascular growth, allows movement of fluid to minimize infection, and reduces edema. NPWT systems consist of a polyurethane foam sponge, semiocclusive adhesive cover, fluid collection system, and a suction pump. The V.A.C. Instill Therapy System combines the benefits of NPWT with instillation to help promote wound healing by automatically delivering a variety of instillation fluids into infected wounds. NPWT sponges are either black or silver and are to be changed every 3 to 7 days.

Indications for NPWT

- Cavitary defects
- Skin grafts (to serve as a dressing and splint)
- Open wounds
  - Chronic, acute, traumatic, dehisced wounds
  - Flaps and grafts

Contraindications for NPWT

- Exposed vessels
- Surgical anastomosis
- Malignancy
- Nonenteric and unexplored fistulas
- Necrotic wounds with eschar

Fast Facts

A complete product guide for wound care products, medical supplies, wound care-related software, and durable medical equipment can be found at:

www.woundsource.com or www.healthproductsforyou.com

Bibliography

Ghomi, E. R., Khalili, S., Khorasani, S. N., Neisiany, R. E., & Ramakrishna, S. (2019, March 18). Wound dressings: Current advances and future directions. *Journal of Applied Polymer Science, 136*(27), 1–2. https://doi.org/10.1002/app.47738

HDFY. Retrieved from www.healthproductsforyou.com

Wound Source. Retrieved from www.woundsource.com

Wound Source Practice Accelerators blog (2018, May 31). Dressing selection: Which dressing to choose? Retrieved from https://www.woundsource.com/blog/dressing-selection-which-dressing-choose

Wound Source Practice Accelerators blog (2018, May 31). Product know-how: The different types of wound care dressings. Retrieved from https://www.woundsource.com/blog/product-know-how-different-types-wound-care-dressings

10

Biologic Agents and Skin Substitutes

INTRODUCTION

The objective of wound healing is to create an environment that minimizes infection, provides the optimal balance of moisture, and facilitates re-epithelialization. In the past, most wound dressings were designed to protect the wound, assist with managing exudate, or provide hydration. Recent advances in wound healing include the introduction of biologic wound products and enhancements in human and synthetic skin substitutes. Skin substitutes aid in wound closure more rapidly by replacing functions of the skin. Biologic agents promote wound closure by inducing natural biochemical processes associated with wound healing. The result is dermal regeneration and re-epithelialization instead of scar tissue formation. It is important for wound care specialist to be familiar with the various biologic and skin substitute agents available and to understand their role in providing either temporary or permanent solutions for wound closure.

In this chapter, you will learn:

1. How biologic agents and skin substitutes facilitate wound closure.
2. The classifications of skin substitutes.
3. The types of biologic agents and skin substitutes available for wound care.

WHAT EXACTLY ARE THEY?

Biologic wound dressings are available in many forms such as gels, powders, solutions, and sheets and are made of natural sources such as collagen, hyaluronan, human keratinocytes, and fibroblasts. These skin substitutes are embedded with live cells and the extracellular matrix (ECM), proteins, and growth factors necessary to regenerate skin and tissue. Bioengineered skin substitutes facilitate healing by initiating biochemical cues that restore normal skin architecture. They assist wound closure through constructive remodeling rather than the formation of scar tissue.

Bioengineered skin substitutes are indicated for a variety of acute wounds as well as chronic, nonhealing wounds and full-thickness or deep-partial thickness burns.

The Five Classifications of Biologic Agents

Cultured Epithelial Autografts (CEAs)

- A large area of keratinocytes is obtained from a small biopsy of healthy skin, cultured, expanded onto larger sheets, ready for application in 3 weeks.
- Indicated for large total body surface area full-thickness burns when limited area is available for donor sites.

Human Skin Allografts (Cadaver Skin)

- Indicated for temporary coverage with partial-thickness burns and a variety of wounds and for wound bed preparation for subsequent autografts (graft using patient's own skin).
- Promotes vascularization, angiogenesis, enhanced capillary growth, and epithelialization in the wound bed.

Allogenic (From the Same Species)

- Derived from human neonatal fibroblasts.
- Collected from placentae of screened donors then preserved onto a variety of forms for application.

Composite

- Derived from human keratinocytes, fibroblasts, and bovine or porcine collagen.
- Available in many different forms
- Indicated for various partial- and full-thickness wounds.

Xenografts

- Acellular derived from porcine or bovine collagen.
- Skin substitutes harvested from animals for use as temporary wound coverage and skin grafts.
- Indicated for partial-thickness burns.

Fast Facts

To prevent waste of valuable biologic agents and skin substitutes, choose products that are available in a range of sizes that can conform to various wound sizes.

Advantages of Biologic Dressings and Skin Substitutes

- Dressings can often stay intact for up to a week resulting in less need for wound care.
- Comfortable and well-tolerated by patients
- Less pain with wound care and dressing changes
- Minimize contamination/infection
- More rapid healing time
- More rapid neovascularization
- Available in a variety of forms and products

Disadvantages of Biologic Dressings and Skin Substitutes

- More expensive than conventional care and dressings
- Learning curve required for proper application techniques and care
- Require meticulous storage and preservation
- Products vary in terms of number of applications needed
- Some require extensive wound preparation
- Medicare coverage varies by region

SKIN SUBSTITUTE PRODUCTS COMMERCIALLY AVAILABLE IN THE UNITED STATES

Affinity® Human Amniotic Allograft

- Affinity is a fresh amniotic membrane aseptically processed and hypothermically preserved.
- Manufacturer: Organogenesis, Inc., Canton, MA, USA.

AlloPatch®

- Allopatch is an aseptically processed human reticular dermal tissue for use as a chronic or acute wound covering.
- Manufacturer: Musculoskeletal Transplant Foundation (dba MTF Biologics), Edison, NJ, USA.

AlloPatch® Pliable

- AlloPatch Pliable is a human reticular dermal tissue.
- Manufacturer: Musculoskeletal Transplant Foundation (dba MTF Biologics).

AlloSkin™ AC Acellular Dermal Matrix

- AlloSkin AC is a meshed, dermis-only human skin graft.
- Manufacturer: AlloSource, Centennial, CO, USA.

AlloSkin™ RT

- AlloSkin RT is a meshed human dermal graft.
- Manufacturer: AlloSource, Centennial, CO, USA.

AlloWrap®

- AlloWrap is a human placental membrane.
- Manufacturer: AlloSource, Centennial, CO, USA.

AltiPlast®

- AltiPlast is a cryopreserved placental matrix derived from human amniotic and chorionic membranes.
- Manufacturer: Aziyo Biologics, Silver Spring, MD, USA.

AltiPly®

- Lyophilized placental membrane.
- Manufacturer: AziyoBiologics, Silver Spring, MD, USA.

AltiPly®
AmnioBand® Allograft Placental Matrix

- AmnioBand is an aseptically processed human allograft placental matrix composed of amnion and chorion for use as an acute or chronic wound covering.
- Manufacturer: Musculoskeletal Transplant Foundation (dba MTF Biologics).

Amnioexcel®

- Amnioexcel is dehydrated human amnion-derived tissue allograft with intact ECM.
- Manufacturer: Integra LifeSciences Corp., Plainsboro, NJ, USA.

AmnioFill® Human Placental Tissue Allograft

- AmnioFill is a nonviable cellular tissue matrix allograft derived from human placental tissue.
- Manufacturer: MiMedx Group, Inc., Marietta, GA, USA.

AmnioFix® Amnion/Chorion Membrane Allograft

- AmnioFix is an allograft composed of dehydrated human amnion/chorion membrane.
- Manufacturer: MiMedx Group, Inc., Marietta, GA, USA.

Amniomatrix® Human Amniotic Suspension Allograft

- Amnionmatrix is a cryopreserved suspension allograft derived from the amniotic membrane and components of the amniotic fluid.
- Manufacturer: Integra LifeSciences, Plainsboro, NJ, USA.

Apligraf®

- Apligraf is a living, bilayered skin substitute. The lower dermal layer combines bovine type I collagen and human fibroblasts (dermal cells). The upper epidermal layer is formed by human keratinocytes (epidermal cells).
- Manufacturer: Organogenesis, Inc., Canton, MA, USA.

Architect® Stabilized Collagen Matrix

- Architect is made from decellularized equine pericardial tissue.
- Manufacturer: Harbor MedTech, Inc., Irvine, CA, USA.

Artacent® Wound

- Wound-specific, dual-layered amniotic tissue graft designed for enhanced efficacy and ease of use. Intended for chronic wounds.
- Manufacturer: Tides Medical, Lafayette, LA, USA.

Bio-ConneKt® Wound Matrix

- The Bio-ConneKt Wound Matrix is composed of reconstituted type I collagen derived from equine tendon.
- Manufacturer: MLM Biologics, Inc., Alachua, FL, USA.

BioDFactor® Viable Tissue Matrix

- BioDFactor Viable Tissue Matrix is a flowable tissue allograft derived from morselized amniotic tissue and components of amniotic fluid.
- Manufacturer: Integra LifeSciences, Plainsboro, NJ, USA.

BioDFence®

- BioDFence G3 and BioDDryFlex are membrane allografts derived from human placental tissues.
- Manufacturer: Integra LifeSciences, Plainsboro, NJ, USA.

Biovance® Amniotic Membrane Allograft

- Biovance is a decellularized, dehydrated human placental membrane with a preserved natural epithelial basement membrane and an intact ECM structure.
- Manufacturer: Alliqua Biomedical, Langhorne, PA, USA.

Cellesta™ Amniotic Membrane

- Cellesta Amniotic Membrane is a placental allograft product. The single-layered allografts are affixed to a polymesh backing and can be sutured, glued, or laid over the desired tissue.
- Manufacturer: Ventris Medical, Newport Beach, CA, USA.

CollaWound Collagen Sponge

- CollWound dressing is composed of cross-linked porous collagen matrix.
- Manufacturer: Collamatrix Co., Ltd., Miaoli County, Taiwan.

Coll-e-derm™

- Coll-e-derm is derived from human placental membrane.
- Manufacturer: Parametrics Medical, Leander, TX, USA.

Cygnus® Amnion Patch Allografts

- Cygnus is derived from human placental membrane.
- Manufacturer: Vivex Biomedical, Atlanta, GA, USA.

Cytal® Wound Matrix

- Cytal is composed of porcine urinary bladder matrix with an intact epithelial basement membrane.
- Manufacturer: Acell, Inc., Columbia, MD, USA.

DermACELL® Human Acellular Dermal Matrix

- DermACELL is a human acellular dermal matrix. DermACELL AWM is intended for chronic wounds.
- Manufacturer: LifeNet Health, Virginia Beach, VA, USA.

Dermagraft®

- Dermagraft is a cryopreserved human fibroblast-derived dermal substitute composed of fibroblasts, ECM, and a bioabsorbable scaffold.
- Manufacturer: Organogenesis, Canton, MA, USA.

Dermapure®

- Dermapure is a decellularized human dermis product.
- Manufacturer: Tissue Regenix Group, San Antonio, TX, USA.

DermaSpan™ Acellular Dermal Matrix

- DermaSpan Acellular Dermal Matrix is derived from allograft human skin.
- Manufacturer: Zimmer Biomet (Biomet Orthopedics), Warsaw, IN, USA.

Dermavest® and Plurivest® Human Placental Connective Tissue Matrix

- Dermavest Human Placental Tissue Matrix is composed of human placental tissue.
- Manufacturer: Aedicell, Inc., Honcoye Falls, NY, USA.

Endoform™ Dermal Template

- Endoform Dermal Template contains a naturally derived bovine collagen ECM that is terminally sterilized.
- Manufacturer: Hollister Wound Care, Libertyville, IL, USA.

EpiCord®

- EpiCord is a dehydrated, nonviable cellular umbilical cord allograft.
- Manufacturer: MiMedx, Inc., Marietta, GA, USA.

Epifix®

- Epifix is a dehydrated human amnion/chorion membrane allograft.
- Manufacturer: MiMedx, Inc., Marietta, GA, USA.

Excellagen®

- Excellagen is collagen gel composed of formulated 2.6% fibrillar bovine dermal collagen (type 1) that is topically applied to the wound surface.
- Manufacturer: Taxus Cardium Pharmaceuticals Group, San Diego, CA, USA.

EZ Derm®

- EZ Derm is a porcine xenograft for partial skin loss injuries or as a temporary cover.
- Manufacturer: Molnlycke Health Care, Norcross, GA, USA.

FloGraft® Amniotic Fluid-Derived Allograft

- FloGraft is chorion-free allograft composed of amnion and amniotic fluid derived from prescreened, live, healthy donors.
- Manufacturer: Applied Biologics, Scottsdale, AZ, USA.

FlowerAmnioPatch™ and Flower AmnioFlo™

- FlowerAmnioPatch is a dual-layer amniotic membrane allograft. FlowerAmnioFlo is a flowable amnion tissue allograft.
- Manufacturer: Flower Orthopedics, Horsham, PA, USA.

FlowerDerm™

- FlowerDerm is a meshed dermis-only decellularized human skin graft.
- Manufacturer: Flower Orthopedics, Horsham, PA, USA.

GammaGraft™

- GammaGraft is an irradiated human skin allograft.
- Manufacturer: Promethean LifeSciences, Inc., Pittsburgh, PA, USA.

Geistlich Derma-Gide™

- Derma-Gide is a porcine, porous, resorbable, 3D matrix designed specifically for the management of wounds.
- Manufacturer: Geistlich Pharma North America, Inc., Princeton, NJ, USA.

Genesis Amniotic Membrane

- Genesis Amniotic Membrane is derived from human placental membrane.
- Manufacturer: Genesis Biologics, Anaheim, CA, USA.

Grafix®

- Grafix is a cryopreserved cellular placental membrane.
- Manufacturer: Osiris Therapeutics, Columbia, MD, USA.

GrafixPL Prime®

- GrafixPL Prime is a lyopreserved cellular placental amniotic membrane.
- Manufacturer: Osiris Therapeutics, Columbia, MD, USA.

GraftJacket™ RTM

- GraftJacket Matrix is a human dermal collagen matrix.
- Manufacturer: Wright Medical Group N.V., Memphis, TN, USA.

Helicoll™

- Helicoll is an acellular collagen matrix derived from bovine sources.
- Manufacturer: EnColl Corp., Fremont, CA, USA.

hMatrix® ADM

- hMatrix ADM is an allograft derived from donated human skin.
- Manufacturer: Bacterin International, Inc., Belgrade, MT, USA.

Hyalomatrix® Tissue Reconstruction Matrix

- Hyalomatrix is a nonwoven pad composed of a wound contact layer made of a derivative of hyaluronic acid in fibrous form with an outer layer composed of a semipermeable silicone membrane.
- Manufacturer: Anika Therapeutics, Bedford, MA, USA.

Integra® Bilayer Matrix Wound Dressing

- Integra Bilayer Wound Matrix is composed of a porous matrix of cross-linked bovine tendon collagen and glycosaminoglycan and a semipermeable polysiloxane (silicone layer).
- Manufacturer: Integra LifeSciences.

Integra® BioFix® Amniotic Membrane Allograft

- Integra BioFix and Biofix Plus are human tissue allografts derived from allogeneic dehydrated and decellularized amniotic membrane.
- Manufacturer: Integra LifeSciences, Plainsboro, NJ, USA.

Integra® BioFix® Flow Placental Tissue Matrix Allograft

- Integra BioFix Flow is derived from decellularized particulate human placental connective tissue matrix.
- Manufacturer: Integra LifeSciences, Plainsboro, NJ, USA.

Integra® Dermal Regeneration Template and Integra® Omnigraft Regeneration Template

- Integra Dermal Regeneration Template has two layers: a thin outer layer of silicone and a thick inner matrix layer of pure bovine collagen and glycosaminoglycan.
- Manufacturer: Integra LifeSciences, Plainsboro, NJ, USA.

Integra® Flowable Wound Matrix

- Integra Flowable Wound Matrix is composed of granulated cross-linked bovine tendon collagen and glycosaminoglycan.
- Manufacturer: Integra LifeSciences, Plainsboro, NJ, USA.

Integra® Matrix Wound Dressing (Originally Avagen Wound Dressing)

- Integra Wound Matrix is composed of a porous matrix of cross-linked bovine tendon collagen and glycosaminoglycan.
- Manufacturer: Integra LifeSciences, Plainsboro, NJ, USA.

InteguPly®

- InteguPly is human acellular dermis.
- Manufacturer: Aziyo Biologics, Silver Springer, MD.

Interfyl™ Human Connective Tissue Matrix

- Interfyl is connective tissue matrix derived from human placenta.
- Manufacturer: Alliqua Biomedical, Langhorne, PA, USA.

Matrix HD® Allograft

- Matrix HD Allograft is an acellular human dermis allograft.
- Manufacturer: RTI Surgical, Alachua, FL, USA.

MicroMatrix®

- MicroMatrix is composed of a porcine-derived extracellular urinary bladder matrix.
- Manufacturer: Acell, Columbia, MD.

Miroderm®

- Miroderm is a noncross-linked acellular wound matrix derived from porcine liver.
- Manufacturer: Miromatrix Medical, Inc., Eden Prairie, MN, USA.

Neox® Wound Allografts

- Neox Wound Matrix is preserved human umbilical cord and amniotic membrane.
- Manufacturer: Amniox Medical, Inc., Miami, FL, USA.

NuShield®

- NuShield is a dehydrated placental allograft.
- Manufacturer: Organogenesis, Inc., Canton, MA.

Ologen™ Collagen Matrix

- Ologen Collagen Matrix is made of cross-linked lyophilized porcine type 1 atelocollagen and glycosaminoglycans.
- Manufacturer: Aeon Astron Europe B.V., Taipei City, Taiwan.

Omega3 Wound (Originally Merigen Wound Dressing)

- Kerecis MariGen Wound Dressing is processed fish dermal matrix composed of fish collagen and is supplied as a sterile intact or meshed sheet.
- Manufacturer: Kerecis, Arlington, VA, USA.

Oasis® Wound Matrix

- Oasis Matrix products are naturally derived scaffolds of ECM, composed of porcine small intestinal submucosa.
- Manufacturer: Smith & Nephew, Inc., Fort Worth, TX, USA.

PalinGen® Membrane and Hydromembrane

- PalinGen Membrane and Hydromembrane are human allografts processed from healthy placental tissue.
- Manufacturer: Amnio Technology, LLC, Phoenix, AZ, USA.

PriMatrix® Dermal Repair Scaffold

- PriMatrix Dermal Repair Scaffold is derived from fetal bovine dermis.
- Manufacturer: Integra LifeSciences, Plainsboro, NJ, USA.

Puracol® and Puracol® Plus Collagen Wound Dressings

- Composed of 100% bovine collagen.
- Manufacturer: Medline Industries, Northfield, IL, USA.

PuraPly® Antimicrobial (PuraPly AM) Wound Matrix (formally called FortaDerm)

- PuraPly Antimicrobial Wound Matrix consists of a collagen sheet collagen with polyhexmethylenebiguanide hydrochloride.
- Manufacturer: Organogenesis, Inc., Canton, MA.

Restorigin™ Amniotic Tissue Patches

- Restorigin Amniotic Tissue Patches are derived from human placenta.
- Manufacturer: Parametrics Medical, Leander, TX, USA.

Restrata™

- Restrata is a fully synthetic electrospun wound dressing composed of randomly oriented nanofibers.
- Manufacturer: Acera Surgical, Inc., St. Louis, MO, USA.

Revita®

- Revita is an intact human placental membrane autograft.
- Manufacturer: StimLabs, LLC, Roswell, GA, USA.

SkinTE™

- SkinTE is an entirely autologous product derived from a sample of the patient's skin.
- Manufacturer: PolarityTE, Salt Lake City, UT, USA.

Talymed®

- Talymed advanced matrix is composed of shortened fibers of poly-N-acetyl glucosamine isolated from microalgae.
- Manufacturer: Marine Polymer Technologies, Inc., Burlington, MA, USA.

TheraForm™ Standard/Sheet Absorbable Collagen Membrane

- TheraForm is a sterile, pliable, porous scaffold made of biocollagen.
- Manufacturer: Sewon Cellontech Co., Seoul, Korea.

TheraSkin®

- TheraSkin is a human, living, split-thickness allograft.
- Manufacturer: LifeNet Health, Solsys Medical, Newport News, VA, USA.

WoundEx® Membrane and WoundEx Flow

- WoundEx Membrane is a dehydrated amniotic membrane. WoundEx Flow is a flowable human placental connective tissue matrix.
- Manufacturer: Skye Biologics, Inc., El Segundo, CA, USA.

Xwrap® Amniotic Membrane-Derived Allograft

- Xwrap is a chorion-free membrane wrap, cover, or patch.
- Manufacturer: Applied Biologics, Scottsdale, AZ, USA.

Bibliography

NCBI Bookshelf. A service of the National Library of Medicine, National Institutes of Health.

Snyder, D. L., Sullivan, M., Margolis, D. J., & Schoelles, K. (February 2020). Skin substitutes for treating chronic wounds. Technical Brief. Agency for Healthcare and Quality. Retrieved from https://www.ncbi.nlm.nih.gov/books/NBK554222/table/ch4.tab1/?report=objectonly

Turner, N., & Badylak, S. (2015, August). The use of biologic scaffolds in the treatment of chronic nonhealing wounds. *Advances in Wound Care, 4*(8), 490–500. http://dx.doi.org/10.1089/wound.2014.0604

Varnado, M. (2020, July 24). Skin substitutes: Understanding product differences. Wound Care Advisor blog. Retrieved from https://woundcareadvisor.com/skin-substitutes-understanding-product-differences/

11

Wound Debridement

INTRODUCTION

Wound debridement is effective in reducing the bioburden of a wound, in controlling and/or preventing wound infection, and in removing necrotic tissue such as eschar or slough. There are several types of wound debridement, one or more of which may be used to access healthy underlying tissue and to interrupt the vicious chronic wound cycle. Debridement choices can range from sharp, autolytic, enzymatic, and mechanical to biodebridement. Wound care practitioners must be familiar with the advantages and disadvantages of these debridement approaches.

In this chapter, you will learn:

1. Indications for debridement and how it facilitates wound healing.
2. The types of gangrene and the importance of not removing dry gangrene.
3. The methods of debridement, how they are classified, and their mechanism of action.
4. How to choose the most suitable debridement method based on advantages and disadvantages.

INDICATIONS FOR WOUND DEBRIDEMENT

Debridement is indicated for any wound covered with devitalized, necrotic tissue such as eschar or slough. Wounds that contain necrotic tissue will not heal. Debridement is also indicated if the wound contains a foreign body or shows signs of infection. The goal for debridement is to promote re-epithelialization by removing bio-film/bioburden and senescent cells. Necrotic tissue impairs wound healing by:

- Preventing angiogenesis (the development of new blood vessels).
- Preventing re-epithelialization (the resurfacing of a wound with epithelium).
- Preventing topical agents from contacting the wound.
- Preventing granulation tissue formation.
- Preventing normal extracellular matrix formation.
- Masking potential underlying infections.
- Preventing the clinician from making an accurate assessment of the wound.

Eschar

Eschar is dead tissue and has the following characteristics:

- Thick and/or leathery appearance
- Brown/black in color
- May be firmly attached or loosely adherent
- Hard or soft
- Wet or dry

Slough

Slough is the moist, devitalized tissue and has the following characteristics:

- Cream/yellow/tan in color
- May be firmly attached or loosely adherent
- May appear slimy, gelatinous, fibrinous, or liquefying
- Made of proteinaceous tissue, fibrin, neutrophils, and bacteria

Gangrene

Gangrene is dead tissue resulting from lack of blood flow to the tissue. See Table 11.1.

Signs and Symptoms of Gangrene

- Skin discoloration: pale, blue (cyanotic), purple (violaceous), black, red
- Edema (swelling) and blister formation with skin sloughing
- A clear line of demarcation (area between healthy and infected skin/tissue)

Table 11.1

	Six Types of Gangrene
Gangrene Type	**Description**
Dry gangrene	Appears dry and black
	Not infected
	Progresses slowly and demarcates (separates) eventually
	Also known as stable eschar
Wet gangrene	Wet appearing eschar
	Acutely infected
Gas gangrene	Wet gangrene
	Most commonly caused by an infection with the bacteria *Clostridium perfringens*
	Produces toxins that release gas that causes extensive tissue death
Internal gangrene	Gangrene that affects one or more internal organs due to blood flow blockages
Fournier's gangrene	Caused by an infection in the genital organs
Progressive bacterial synergistic gangrene	Rare type of gangrene that causes painful skin lesions following surgery
	Also known as Meleney's gangrene

- Sudden, severe pain
- Foul-smelling drainage from site of infected tissue
- General malaise (not feeling well)
- Low blood pressure
- High fever
- Rapid heart rate (tachycardia)
- Feeling lightheaded
- Shortness of breath
- Altered mental status or confusion.

Treatment for Gangrene

Treatment strategies for dry gangrene include keeping the affected area dry and protected. Effective management of wet gangrene, gas gangrene, Fournier's gangrene, and internal gangrene includes surgical debridement (excision) of the infected tissue and/or amputation, as well as broad-spectrum antibiotics and intensive medical management related to sepsis.

TYPES OF DEBRIDEMENT

Sharp Debridement

Sharp Selective Debridement

- The wound care specialist removes loosely adherent, nonviable tissue using scissors and forceps ("pick-ups").
- In most states, selective debridement falls within the nurse's scope of practice.

Sharp Surgical Debridement

- Usually performed in the operating room by a physician or mid-level provider.
- Includes excision of large amounts of nonviable tissue.

Laser Debridement

- Uses a CO_2 laser for controlled removal of nonviable tissue.
- The type of laser and number of passes determines the depth of tissue removed and is beneficial in that debridement can be precisely controlled.

Waterjet Hydrosurgery

- Jets of high-pressure water or other solutions precisely target nonviable tissue while aspirating debris at the same time.

Fast Facts

Contraindications for Debridement
1. Clean wounds without slough or necrotic tissue.
2. Dry, stable, black eschar on pressure ulcers that show no signs or symptoms of infection (Agency for Health Care Policy and Research, 1994).
3. Dry, stable, ischemic wounds resulting from peripheral arterial disease or certain autoimmune conditions.

Advantages of Sharp Debridement

- A highly effective, quick method to remove dead tissue.
- Can be combined with other debridement methods.
- Can be performed in a variety of clinical settings.

Disadvantages of Sharp Debridement

- Sharp debridement can initiate bleeding, so take caution with patients who are receiving anticoagulant therapy or have bleeding disorders.
- Avoid introducing transient bacteremia from infected wounds during sharp debridement.
- Sharp surgical and waterjet debridement are more costly procedures.
- Clinicians must have the skill level to perform sharp debridement.
- Healing can be delayed if adjacent healthy tissue is damaged.

Autolytic Debridement

Autolytic debridement is considered selective debridement in that only the necrotic tissue is liquified by the body's own enzymes while healthy tissue is spared. Wound exudate accumulates under semiocclusive or occlusive dressings. This fluid accumulation causes the body's own enzymes and moisture to rehydrate, soften, and liquefy eschar and/or slough.

This debridement is recommended for clean wounds with only a small amount of necrotic tissue. As the necrotic tissue breaks down, the wound bed appears larger in size; however, this does not mean that the wound is infected or the dressing is ineffective.

Success of the debridement should be clearly observable within 3 to 4 days. Autolytic debridement is a good choice when anticoagulant therapy renders sharp surgical debridement unfeasible.

Agents available to assist with autolytic include:

- Hydrogel-Skintegrity (Medline)
- Plurogel (Medline)
- Medihoney (Derma Sciences)
- Hydrocolloids
- Highly absorptive dressings

Advantages of Autolytic Debridement

- Can be used alone or in conjunction with other debridement techniques.
- Safe, easy, and painless
- Inexpensive

Disadvantages of Autolytic Debridement

- Autolysis is a slow process.
- Requires close assessment as autolysis can promote anaerobic bacterial growth and infection.
- Periwound needs to be protected with skin barrier.
- Requires daily dressing changes or more frequently for heavy exudate.

Enzymatic Debridement

Enzymatic debridement utilizes enzymatic agents to accelerate degradation of nonviable tissue. The only FDA-approved enzymatic ointment is Collagenase (Santyl). Collagenase (Smith & Nephew) is derived from the bacterium *Clostridium histolyticum* and produces selective debridement by breaking down collagen.

Advantages of Enzymatic Debridement

- Can be used alone or in conjunction with other debridement techniques.
- Safe and easy to apply.
- Minimally painful

Disadvantages of Enzymatic Debridement

- Eschar may require cross-hatching with a scalpel for the product to penetrate the dead tissue.
- Most effective if applied 2 to 3 times a day.
- Santyl is expensive.
- Heavy metal or ionized silver products can deactivate the ointments.

Fast Facts

Selective debridement means that only nonviable tissue is targeted. Nonselective debridement means that both nonviable and healthy tissue can be targeted.

Always provide diligent wound and skin assessment if using a nonselective debridement method.

Biodebridement

Biodebridement is a "prescription only" FDA-approved medical intervention for wound debridement that utilizes sterile fly maggot therapy to break down and ingest infected or necrotic tissue. Typically, about 10 maggots per square inch of necrotic tissue are used. The maggots are kept in the wound for 72 hours using a protective dressing outlined with a hydrocolloid base (BioBag), then removed and discarded.

Advantages of Biodebridement

- Safe and effective
- Relatively inexpensive
- Does not damage healthy tissue (selective debridement)

Disadvantages of Biodebridement

- Maggots must be used within 12 hours of receipt.
- Patient education: "The yuck factor"
- Learning curve for successful application and use
- Lack of availability: The largest producer of medicinal maggots closed its American laboratory in 2019 due to lack of profitability.
- Insurance reimbursement can be problematic as no maggot-specific Current Procedural Terminology (CPT) code exists.

Wet-to-Dry Mechanical Debridement

Broadly, mechanical debridement is nonselective and involves using solutions, wound cleansers, and scrubs to remove fibrous slough and eschar. Sharp debridement with scissors or forceps, irrigation, and hydrotherapy is also considered a form of mechanical debridement.

Wet-to-dry dressings are considered a form of mechanical debridement and involve wetting a dressing with specific solutions and allowing them to dry, thus providing debridement once removed from the wound bed.

Common solutions used for mechanical wet-to-dry debridement include:

- Sodium hypochlorite (basic dakins)
- Puracyn
- Normal saline

Advantages of Mechanical Wet-to-Dry Debridement

- Relatively inexpensive
- Easy to administer
- Useful for large wounds or cavities
- Can control odor
- Can control infection
- Can be used with other debridement types

Disadvantages of Mechanical Wet-to-Dry Debridement

- Can be painful, therefore, requires premedication
- Nonselective in nature
- Indicated for short-term treatment
- Length of time required to promote wound healing
- Not useful for intact eschar.

Irrigation

Irrigation debridement utilizes equipment that combines a pulsating irrigation fluid with suction. Treatments usually take 15 to 30 minutes and are most effective if performed twice daily at a pressure range from 4 to 15 psi.

- High-pressure irrigation delivers pressure of 8 to 12 psi; for example, a 35 mL syringe with a large bore angiocatheter.
- Pulsatile high-pressure lavage provides intermittent high-pressure irrigation combined with suction. The pressure may be adjusted.

Fast Facts

A bulb syringe delivers a psi of only 4 (or less) and is not sufficient to remove eschar and slough from a wound bed. Check the effectiveness of your wound cleanser spray. The psi should be noted on the bottle.

Advantages of Irrigation Debridement

- Provides effective debridement
- Has been shown to improve granulation tissue growth
- Easy to perform

Disadvantages of Irrigation Debridement

- Has the potential for dissemination of bacteria from the spray
- Requires protective gear
- Supplies may be costly
- Process can be time-consuming
- Not recommended for patients on anticoagulant therapy

Hydrotherapy Debridement

Hydrotherapy involves cleaning and removal of necrotic debris by immersion in specialty tanks, showering, or spraying. It is indicated for patients who need aggressive cleaning or softening of necrotic tissue.

Advantages of Hydrotherapy Debridement

- It is an effective debridement method for large surface areas, the loosening of adherent necrotic tissue, and dressings.

Disadvantages of Hydrotherapy Debridement

- Can cause periwound maceration.
- Can put the patient at risk for water-borne infection if the equipment is not properly sanitized.
- Increases risk of cross-contamination among patients.

Bibliography

Hadi, S., & Inwood, R. (2016, December). Current and emerging debridement options in wound care. *Podiatry Today, 29*(12), 46–51. Retrieved from https://www.podiatrytoday.com/current-and-emerging-debridement-options-wound-care

Manna, B., & Morrison, C. (2020, February 14). Wound debridement. NCBI Bookshelf; A service of the National Library of Medicine, National Institutes of Health. Retrieved from from https://www.ncbi.nlm.nih.gov/books/NBK507882/

Mayo Clinic; Gangrene. Retrieved from https://www.mayoclinic.org/diseases-conditions/gangrene/symptoms-causes/syc-20352567

Sherman, R. (2019, June 20). Maggot debridement therapy in the United States. Ron Sherman's blog. Retrieved from https://www.woundsource.com/blog/maggot-debridement-therapy-in-united-states#:~:text=Medicinal%20maggots%20are%20widely%20acknowledged,of%20patients%20scheduled%20for%20amputation

12

Hyperbaric Oxygen Therapy

INTRODUCTION

A good physician treats the disease, the great physician treats the patient who has the disease.

-Unknown

Hyperbaric oxygen therapy (HBOT) is a valuable adjunctive therapy for certain types of wounds. In the 1930s, the military developed and tested HBOT for deep-sea diving and aeronautics. Clinical trials are ongoing to find more uses for HBOT. HBOT can be performed as an outpatient procedure or initiated if the patient is hospitalized. Be familiar with the indications for HBOT since early recognition and initiation of therapy can make a significant difference in the outcome for the patient.

In this chapter, you will learn:

1. The definitions of and indications for HBOT.
2. The advantages of and contraindications for HBOT.

HYPERBARIC OXYGEN THERAPY

The term *hyperbaric* literally means higher pressure. HBOT is the breathing of 100% oxygen in a monochamber or multiperson chamber, which delivers pressures of 2.0 to 2.4 times the normal atmospheric pressure. This therapy has various potential mechanisms of action, including increasing partial pressure of oxygen in the tissues of the body to a degree several times greater than that which can be achieved through normal atmospheric pressure. In addition to its effects on cellular function, HBOT impacts the immune system. Oxygen has an antimicrobial effect, especially in anaerobic infections. HBOT stimulates phagocytosis, benefits fibroblast activity, and promotes angiogenesis.

The number of treatments varies depending on the patient's diagnosis but generally ranges from two to three for carbon monoxide poisoning and decompression sickness to upward of 20 to 40 for nonhealing wounds. The average treatment time is 110 minutes: 10 minutes to reach appropriate pressure, 90 minutes at pressure, and 10 minutes to return to normal pressure.

Indications for HBOT

- Acute carbon monoxide intoxication
- Decompression illness
- Gas embolism
- Gas gangrene
- Peripheral ischemia
- Crush injuries and severed limbs
- Necrotizing soft-tissue infections
- Cyanide poisoning
- Osteoradionecrosis and soft-tissue radionecrosis
- Actinomycosis
- Compromised skin grafts and flaps
- Certain diabetic lower extremity wounds
- Refractory osteomyelitis

Risks of HBOT

HBOT is generally a safe procedure. A certified physician or other healthcare provider is present with the patient throughout the treatments. Potential risks involved with HBOT include:

- Temporary nearsightedness caused by eye lens changes
- Ear pain secondary to middle ear trauma
- Collapsed lung (barotrauma)
- Seizures secondary to oxygen toxicity
- Confinement anxiety
- Fire due to the oxygen-rich environment

Contraindications to HBOT

Conditions that necessitate precautions but are not necessarily a complete contraindication are:

- History of spontaneous pneumothorax
- Severe sinus infection
- Upper respiratory infection
- Asymptomatic pulmonary lesions on chest x-ray
- High fever (greater than 39C)
- History of ear or chest surgery
- Congenital spherocytosis (shortage of red blood cells)
- Anemias or blood disorders
- Seizure disorder
- Optic neuritis or sudden blindness
- Middle ear infection
- Uncontrolled diabetes
- Pregnancy
- COPD/emphysema
- Implanted pacemakers: Call the manufacturer of device for clarification of safety
- Internal cardiac defibrillators (ICDs): Should be deactivated before treatment and reactivated after decompression.

Fast Facts

Untreated pneumothorax is an absolute contraindication for HBOT.

PATIENT EDUCATION TO PREVENT COMPLICATIONS

- Teach air-equalization techniques to prevent ear pressure by yawning or swallowing.
- Instruct patient not to:
  - Hold their breath
  - Wear cosmetics, contact lenses, hairspray, perfumes, or lip balm to the treatment since these products can be combustible.
- Before starting HBOT:
  - Remove all petroleum-based dressings before the treatment. These products can be combustible.
  - Assess for anxiety and blood sugar fluctuations.
- HBOT physicians can prescribe medications and/or nasal sprays to control anxiety and limit ear pressure and pain.

Fast Facts

Resources for Hyperbaric Oxygen Therapy Certification
National Board of Diving and Hyperbaric Medical Technology: www.nbdhmt.org
Undersea and Hyperbaric Medical Society: www.uhms.org
Baromedical Nurses Association: www.hyperbaricnurses.org

Bibliography

Clair, D. (August 6, 2020). Hyperbaric oxygen therapy as an adjunct therapy for wound care. Wound Care Advisor. Retrieved from https://woundcareadvisor.com/hyperbaric-oxygen-therapy-adjunct-therapy-wound-care/

Hyperbaric oxygen therapy indications, contraindications, and complications. Retrieved from https://hyperbaricoxygentherapy.com/PDFs/contraindications.pdf

13

Caring for Ostomies and Fistulas

INTRODUCTION

Even dedicated, experienced, and specialized nurses in the field of ostomy management find the artificial openings and abnormal passageways of ostomies and fistulas overwhelming at times. Caring for ostomies and fistulas is a multifaceted, complex process. Every ostomy and fistula is as unique as the patient of whom it is a part. For the wound care specialist who seeks to expand their realm of expertise, it takes willingness and time to develop an expert knowledge base for the care of ostomies and fistulas. This chapter provides information about ostomies and fistulas that will encourage knowledge growth and enhance the expertise of the dedicated wound care specialist.

In this chapter, you will learn:

1. The different etiologies of ostomies and fistulas and some common complications.
2. The classification of ostomies and fistulas by location and complexity.
3. The types of products that are used in the care of ostomies and fistulas and how to use them, nutritional management, and methods of odor control.

OSTOMIES

An ostomy is a surgical opening in the abdomen for the elimination of body wastes. An incision is made through the abdominal wall. The end of the bowel is pulled through the opening, which is then called a stoma. Stomas are not painful. Where the opening is made and how much of the intestine or bladder is removed dictate the kind of ostomy. See Table 13.1.

Colostomy

- Can be temporary or permanent.
- Involves an opening in the large intestine (colon) for the elimination of stools. Loss of rectum usually involves a permanent colostomy.
- After healing, stools are semiformed to formed and brown in color.

Ileostomy

- Can be temporary or permanent.
- Involves an opening in the small intestine to bypass the colon for the elimination of stools. The temporary alternative method is removal of the colon and rectum, creating an internal pouch from the small intestine to hold stools, and attaching the pouch to the anus (ileoanal reservoir).
- Stools are green liquid at first, and later become semiformed and brownish.

Urostomy

- A permanent bladder replacement for holding urine.
- An ileal loop or colon conduit is performed using the end section of the small intestine (ileum) or the beginning of the large intestine (cecum) to form a stoma for urine to pass through.

Table 13.1

Colostomy Classification and Stoma Sites		
Colostomy Type	**Stoma Location**	**Output Description**
Ascending colostomy	Usually on the right side	Liquid or pasty
Transverse colostomy	Usually in the middle	Semisolid with odor
Descending colostomy	Usually on the left side	Normal in appearance with odor
Sigmoid colostomy	Usually on the left side	Normal in appearance with odor
Ileostomy	Usually on the lower right side	Liquid or paste-like

Stoma Assessment

Healthy, well-perfused stomas are bright red. New stomas are edematous and will shrink in time. A pink stoma can be indicative of anemia. Gray or black stomas indicate compromised blood flow to the bowel. Although the stoma itself is moist, the surrounding skin should be clean, dry, and intact.

Stoma Measurement

The stoma should be measured with each pouch change. A template can be made from the wafer backing and used to cut future pouches. The wafer should be no more than 1/8 of an inch larger than the stoma. Good hygiene and skin care are essential for ostomy appliances to be effective.

Common Stoma Complications

Ideally, stomas should be marked by a wound, ostomy, and continence nurse (WOCN) or the surgeon before surgery. Common post-surgery stoma complications include:

Poor Site

- When the stoma location has been surgically placed in the belt line, is too close to a bony prominence or the umbilicus, or is in skin creases, it makes management and pouching difficult.

Hernias

- Common with ostomies because the opening is made through the muscle to bring the stoma to the skin surface.
- Tend to recur.

Stoma Necrosis

- Tissue death from poor circulation and compromised blood flow.
- Stoma will start to appear dark red or violaceous, progressing to black.

Retraction

- Stoma withdraws back below the level of the skin.

Prolapse

- Bowel expands through the stoma.

Fast Facts

Resources for ostomy certification
www.wcei.net
www.webwocnurse.com
www.nawccb.org

The Pouching System

Ostomy pouches may be a one- or two-piece system. In the two-piece system, a pouch collects waste and a wafer holds the pouch in place. In the one-piece system, a wafer connects to the pouch. There are many varieties of pouches and wafers, but the fewer the products the patient has to use, the better. If there is a problem with the pouch, troubleshoot before using more products. See Table 13.2.

OSTOMY AND FISTULA PRODUCTS

All ostomies require the patient to wear an ostomy pouch for elimination of waste. This is related to the surgery bypassing the sphincter muscle, causing involuntary control of elimination.

Fistulas may be difficult to dress or pouch; however, protecting the skin is crucial. The specialty products listed in Table 13.3 aid in choosing and achieving an effective skin management plan.

Table 13.2

Troubleshooting Pouches and Appliances	
Did you apply warmth and pressure to the wafer?	It takes warmth and gentle pressure to seal the wafer to the skin.
Have you observed the patient's abdomen as they move from a lying to sitting position?	The patient may need a more flexible pouch, such as a one-piece system or a pouch with convexity.
Is the stoma flush or contracted?	You might need a pouch with more convexity.
Does the patient have deep skin folds?	You may need to use ostomy paste or a paste strip for a secure seal.
Can the patient see where the pouch is?	The patient may need to use a mirror.
Is the pouch being emptied regularly?	The seal can break if the pouch becomes too full of stool or gas. A gas filter may be necessary.

Table 13.3

Ostomy and Fistula Products

Product	Actions and Possible Problems
Barrier creams	Protect the skin and repel moisture. If they are oily, the pouch will not seal effectively.
Pastes (tube or strips)	Makes the skin surface level. It acts as caulking for protection but can melt with urine.
Ostomy powder	Absorbs moisture from denuded skin and creates a barrier.
Pouches	These are the containers for effluent, stools, and odor.
Skin barrier sealants and wipes	Provide a smooth layer to allow the pouch to stick over powder, helpful with ileostomies.
Skin barrier rings	Used as a level on concave skin surfaces; can be used in place of paste or to add convexity.
Solid wafers	Used to level the skin surface and to protect skin from effluent. Secure pouches in place.

Ostomy Pouch Guidelines

1. Supplies
   a. Water
   b. Nonsterile gauze
   c. Scissors
   d. Pouch with wafer and pouch closure clip
   e. Pattern
   f. Paste (if needed)
2. Position patient for easy access and remove the pouch.
3. Clean the stoma and surrounding skin.
4. Measure the stoma.
5. Fill in uneven areas with strips or paste.
6. Prepare the wafer by tracing the pattern on paper backing and cutting to fit.
7. Remove the paper backing.
8. Snap the pouch on the ring if using a two-piece system.
9. Apply a ring of paste around the stoma opening on the wafer of the pouch (do not spread the paste) and apply the wafer.
10. Control stoma drainage with gauze.
11. Gently hold the pouch in place, giving it time to conform and seal.
12. Close the bottom edge of the drainable pouch with a clamp or clampless closure device. You may picture-frame the edges of the wafer with paper tape or waterproof tape.

13. Document the procedure, color of stoma, condition of the skin, appearance of elimination, and patient/family education.

14. Have new ostomy patients or their family/care provider assist with the procedure.

Fast Facts

Reimbursement and coverage for ostomy supplies may vary; therefore, always consider the different insurers and regional reimbursement policies.

FISTULAS

A fistula is an abnormal passageway because of communication from an organ in the body through the surface of the skin. An external fistula is named according to the organ from which the drainage originates, such as the small bowel or pancreas. Fistulas are commonly classified as either simple or complex.

- Simple: Short, direct, without associated abscess or other organ involvement.
- Complex:
  - Type 1: Associated with abscess or multiple organs.
  - Type 2: On the surface; often drains through the base of an open wound.

A fistula may also be classified as purposeful if it is created for a specific reason or as inadvertent if it is a complication from disease, trauma, surgery, inflammation, or a congenital defect. See Table 13.4.

Assessing Fistulas

Take your time assessing fistulas. Thorough assessment and documentation will facilitate the best collaborative intervention choices for the patient from a multidisciplinary approach. Important things to document regarding a fistula are:

1. Where is the fistula?
  a. Is it internal or external?
  b. Is it close to an ostomy site, wound, or surgical incision?
  c. Is it near a bony prominence?
  d. Is it in a concave area?
2. Is there more than one?

Table 13.4

Anatomically Based Classification of Fistulas	
Classification	**Description**
Colocutaneous	A passageway between the colon and the skin.
Colovesical	A fistula between the colon and the bladder.
Enterocutaneous	A cutaneous fistula connecting the intestines and the skin.
Rectovaginal	A fistula connecting the rectum and the vagina.
Vesicovaginal	An abnormal connection between the bladder and the vagina.

3. How much is the fistula draining? This is called effluent.
   a. Low volume is considered less than 200 mL/24 hr.
   b. High volume is considered more than 200 mL/24 hr.
   c. Note the color and consistency.
4. Assess the skin surrounding the fistula.
   a. Is the skin intact, denuded, or macerated?
   b. Are there signs of infection?
5. Assess the patient's pain.

Establishing a Plan of Care for Fistulas

Order imaging studies, such as a CT or MRI, to establish the origin of the fistula, the condition of the adjacent organs, and to rule out the possibility of obstruction or abscess. Obtain a thorough patient history and physical to assess for inflammatory bowel diseases such as Crohn's disease, previous radiation therapy, inadequate blood supply, abdominal trauma, tumors, or the presence of a foreign body.

Fistulas require frequent reassessment and aggressive care. Determine if it can be pouched. High-output fistulas are managed better with a pouch instead of a dressing. If pouching is not suitable, suction systems or V.A.C. therapy may be an appropriate option. Suction systems contain the effluent with low, intermittent suction. Consider V.A.C. therapy for the application of direct pressure closure.

Nutritional Factors

- Replace electrolytes lost through the effluent.
- Replace vitamins.
- Rehydrate with IV fluids if necessary.
- Consider total parenteral nutrition (TPN), fat emulsions, and enteral nutrition as needed especially if the patient is NPO.

- Correct anemia with blood products or iron replacement.
- Eliminate foods that cause discomfort for the patient. See Tables 13.5 through 13.8.

   Odor-Reducing Foods

- Buttermilk
- Cranberry juice
- Parsley
- Yogurt

Table 13.5

Gas-Forming Foods		
Fruits and Vegetables	**Animal Products**	**Other**
Asparagus	Dairy products	Beer
Broccoli	Eggs	Carbonated drinks
Brussel sprouts	Fish	Sugars
Cabbage		Sweets
Cucumbers		
Corn		
Dried beans		
Garlic		
Melons		
Radishes		
Spinach		
Sweet potatoes		

Table 13.6

Odor-Producing Foods		
Vegetables	**Animal Products**	**Other**
Asparagus	Chicken	Coffee
Broccoli	Egg	
Brussel sprouts	Fish	
Cabbage	Seafood	
Cauliflower		
Garlic		
Onion		

Table 13.7

Stool-Thickening Foods

Fruits and Vegetables	Animal Products	Carbohydrates	Other
Applesauce	Boiled milk	Bread	Creamy peanut butter
Bananas	Butter	Pasta	Marshmallows
Potatoes	Cheese	Pretzels	Tapioca
		White bread	Tea
		White rice	

Table 13.8

High-Fiber Foods

Vegetables	Fruits	Other
Raw coleslaw	Tomatoes	Coconut
Salad greens	Raw apples	Mushrooms
Celery	Strawberries	Nuts
Cooked spinach	Grapes	Popcorn
Green beans	Pineapple	
Corn		

Foods That Control Mild Constipation

- Cooked fruits and vegetables
- Fruit juices and fluids

Healthcare providers need to consider the psychological aspect of having an ostomy or fistula. Offer support and resources to manage pain, anxiety, body image, and expense of treatment. Get to know your local wound, ostomy, and continence nurses and wound specialists. Most of them are more than willing to offer support and assistance.

WOUND ODORS

Professional Behavior for Managing Wound Odors

Many wounds are accompanied by odors, which may be quite unpleasant. To avoid embarrassing patients in such instances, be prepared to manage wound odors in a professional, compassionate, and empathetic manner.

Strategies to cope with wound odors:

- Wear a mask when performing wound care.
- Use a scent inside the mask such as toothpaste, peppermints, or perfume.
- Avoid behaviors that communicate disrespect; for example, do not comment on wound odors and refrain from wrinkling the nose or making other unpleasant expressions.

Wound Odor Sources

- Wounds with bioburden (e.g., *Clostridium, Proteus, Klebsiella, Pseudomonas*, bacteria)
- Wounds with necrotic tissue, slough/pus
- Drain sites
- Fistulas
- Ostomies
- End-stage wounds (fungating wounds)
- Certain types of dressings or inappropriate dressings (e.g., hydrocolloids)
- Poor hygiene

Effective Wound Odor Control

- Change gauze dressings more frequently for heavily draining wounds or change to a type of odor-controlling dressing.
- Change linens and patient gowns daily or more often as needed.
- Bathe the patient more frequently.
- Remove soiled linens and dressings from the patient's room.
- Use a deodorant for the patient and a room spray that eliminates odors.
- Use the correct size and type of ostomy bag, deodorant, and skin sealant.
- Address the cause of the odor such as debriding wounds and controlling infection.
- Use charcoal-based dressings and/or antimicrobial dressings.

Fast Facts

Helpful Ostomy Organizations
Crohn's and Colitis Foundation of America, Inc.
www.crohnscolitisfoundation.org

International Foundation for Functional Gastrointestinal Disorders
www.iffgd.org

The National Digestive Diseases Clearinghouse
http://digestive.niddk.nih.gov

The Wound, Ostomy, and Continence Nurse Society
www.wocn.org

The United Ostomy Association of America
www.ostomy.org

The Young Ostomate and Diversion Alliance of America
www.uoaa.org

14

The Promotion of Skin Integrity

INTRODUCTION

Why is skin care so important? The skin is the largest organ of the body and performs major functions such as absorption from respiration, control of evaporation, heat regulation, protection from pathogens, sensation, communication, water resistance, and metabolism. By performing these functions, the skin protects the internal structures of the body. The skin's characteristics are constantly changing in response to environmental, chemical, and physical factors such as the sun, age, hydration, nutrition, medications, and skin care products. If the skin's integrity is compromised, a person's well-being may be at risk. Practical assessment, appropriate care, and prevention are the keys to promoting optimum skin care integrity.

In this chapter, you will learn:

1. Factors that affect skin integrity.
2. How to perform a skin assessment.
3. FDA-approved categories and manufacturers of skin care products.
4. Why incontinence maintenance is the foundation of a successful skin and wound care program.

FACTORS THAT AFFECT SKIN INTEGRITY

Aging

- The aging process can decrease all the normal skin functions over time.

Allergies

- Allergies are caused by irritants that can lead to itching, skin rashes, pain, and skin breakdown.

Circulation

- Poor circulation can cause skin breakdown and ulcerations.

Hydration

- Dehydration can cause dry, cracked, scaly skin.
- Lack of fluids, high humidity, age, and lost sebum contribute to skin dehydration.

Lifestyle Habits

- Poor hygiene can cause skin infections.
- Smoking diminishes circulation to the skin.

Medications

- Corticosteroids cause thinning of skin due to interference with collagen synthesis and epidermal regeneration.
- Anticoagulants may cause bruising and trauma.
- Some medications may cause skin sloughing.

Nutrition

- Poor nutrition can cause skin breakdown. A well-balanced diet of proteins, carbohydrates, fats, vitamins, and minerals is essential for healthy skin.
- Patients with skin compromise require increased dietary intake.

Soaps

- Normal bathing restores skin pH. Harsh chemicals in some soaps used over a long period of time can impair the skin's resistance to bacteria and hydration.

Sun Exposure

- Excessive sun exposure decreases skin elasticity, promotes wrinkles, and is a major factor in skin cancer.

SKIN ASSESSMENT

Perform a head-to-toe skin assessment on every patient, paying particular attention to bony prominences and skin folds. A thorough skin assessment can give the healthcare provider realistic indicators of the patient's skin condition, circulation status, and ability to heal. Skin integrity may be difficult and challenging with sick, compromised patients. Performing a basic skin assessment is crucial to implementing appropriate care.

Skin Assessment Indicators

Capillary Refill

■ An indicator of blood perfusion at the capillary level.

Color

■ White, pale, ashy, waxy skin may be an indicator of poor peripheral circulation, frostbite, or a deep burn.
■ Blue- or gray-colored skin indicates cyanosis.
■ Red skin can indicate fever, infection, partial-thickness burns, or carbon monoxide poisoning.
■ Yellow skin may be an indicator of liver disease.

Integrity

■ Check the overall health of the skin.
■ Observing any fragility, bruising, skin tears, excoriation, denuded areas, decreased sensation, edema, wounds, old scars, and healed ulcer sites.

Moisture

■ Excessively dry, clammy, or sticky skin may be an indicator of underlying disease processes.

Poor Hygiene

■ Odors can reflect infection or wounds.

Temperature

■ Healthy skin is warm and dry to touch.
■ Skin that feels hot can be an indicator of fever, hyperthermia, inflammation, or minor burn.
■ Skin that is cold can be an indicator of poor circulation, sepsis, hypothermia, or frostbite.

Turgor

- Normal skin turgor springs back to normal after it has been pinched.
- Decreased skin turgor is an indicator of dehydration.

Fast Facts

Skin Care Products

Are your skin care products approved by the U.S. FDA? As a patient advocate, understand that under federal law, the products you use on your patients may be approved as a cosmetic, drug, soap, or a combination of these. They may not be FDA approved at all. FDA approval ensures that a product has not been adulterated or mis-branded. The FDA categorizes drugs, soaps, and cosmetics by their intended use. There are multiple ways in which the FDA establishes the intended use of a product based on its ingredients by regulating claims on product labels, in advertising, and on the Internet. For more information on the FDA's skin care product approval criteria, see: http://www.fda.gov.

COMMON SKIN CARE FORMULARY OPTIONS

Cleansers

Cleansers are used for bathing and for removing surface dirt, impurities, perspiration, and excessive oils. Bathing with advanced cleansers also helps rehydrate and nourish skin.

Topical Antifungals

Antifungal medications come in a variety of forms such as creams, powders, solutions, or ointments and treat dermatophyte and fungal infections.

Moisturizers

Moisturizers come in different formulations. Understand the differences among lotions, creams, and ointments to choose the most appropriate product for a particular need. See Table 14.1.

Choose skin care products carefully. Skin care integrity is the foundation of a successful wound and skin care program. See Table 14.2.

Table 14.1

Skin Care Products		
Product	**Purpose**	**Characteristics**
Lotions	Good for normal to mildly dry skin	Lotions are made with oils, usually mixed in a low-viscosity water base that is easily absorbed into the skin.
Creams	Good for moderately to very dry skin and to prevent skin cracking or tears	Creams are emulsified oils, usually mixed in a high-viscosity water base.
Ointments	Good for moisture protection and to remove thick, dead skin on heels and feet.	Ointments are very viscous, semisolid preparations and usually have an occlusive oil base. Ointments are good emollients for active ingredients in topicals.
Zinc-oxide barrier	Good as a moisture barrier for excoriated skin resulting from incontinence or other skin irritants.	Zinc-oxide powder is added to an assortment of cream bases.

Table 14.2

Skin Care Products (Not All Inclusive)		
Skin and Incontinence Cleansers		
Bathing Products	**Disposable Bathing Products**	**Incontinence Cleansers**
Remedy 4-in-1 by Medline	ReadyBath by Medline	Aloe Vesta® Foam by ConvaTec
Secura™ by Smith & Nephew	Aloe Vesta® by ConvaTec	Restore® by Hollister
Vashe by Vitality Medical	Attends Washcloths® by 3M	Bedside-Care® by Coloplast
ApriVera® by Derma Sciences	Baza Cleanse & Protect by Coloplast	Coloplast Cleanse & Protect All-in-One Perineal by Coloplast
Gentle Rain® by Coloplast	Comfort Bath® by Sage	Soothe & Cool® by Medline
Septi-Soft® by ConvaTec	TENA Bathing Glove by Essity	Secura™ by Smith & Nephew
Cavilon™ Skin Cleanser by 3M		

(continued)

Table 14.2

Skin Care Products (Not All Inclusive) (*continued*)

Skin and Incontinence Cleansers

Bathing Products	Disposable Bathing Products	Incontinence Cleansers
Remedy by Medline	Remedy by Medline	Remedy by Medline
Micro-Guard® by Coloplast	DermaFungal by DermaRite	MITRAZOL® by Healthpoint
Baza® by Coloplast	Critic-Aid® by Coloplast	Micro-Guard® by Coloplast
INZO™ by Medline	Cardinal Health by Cardinal	Clotrimazole powder
Clotrimazole cream	Clotrimazole ointment	Nystatin powder
Nystatin cream	Nystatin ointment	Miconazole powder
Miconazole cream	Miconazole ointment	Thera Antifungal Body Powder by McKesson
Lotrimin cream	Lotrimin ointment	Lotrimin powder
Lamisil cream	Aloe Vesta® by ConvaTec	Lamisil powder

Moisturizers

Creams	Ointments	Barrier Creams (Zinc Oxide)
Sensi-Care® by ConvaTec	Aloe Vesta® Convatec	Sensi-Care® by ConvaTec
Uni-Derm® by Smith & Nephew	CURAD Vitamin A&D by Medline	Secura™ by Smith & Nephew
Cavilon™ Emollient by 3M	Secura™ by Smith & Nephew	Bacitracin Zinc by Dynarex
Eucerin® by Beiersdorf	Restore® by Hollister	INZO Barrier Cream by Medline
Remedy Intensive Skin Therapy by Medline	Calmoseptine® by Calmoseptine	McKesson Skin Protectant by McKesson
THERA Moisturizing Body Cream by McKesson	Aquaphor® by Beiersdorf	Coloplast Thick by Coloplast
Coloplast Atrac-Tain by Coloplast	Baza® by Coloplast	Calmoseptine® Barrier by Calmoseptine
Coloplast Sween by Coloplast		Critic-Aid Barrier Paste by Coloplast
Pedifix Deep Healing Diabetic Foot Cream by Pedifix		
Secura® by Smith & Nephew		
Beta Glucan Pro by Stellen Medical		

FECAL AND BLADDER INCONTINENCE

According to the National Association for Continence (NAFC), 25 million Americans are affected by either bladder or bowel control issues. Urinary incontinence affects close to 18 million women alone. Despite the high success in treating incontinence issues, only one out of 12 people seek medical treatment. See Table 14.3.

Table 14.3

Types of Incontinence	
Anatomic incontinence	Leakage caused by an anatomic or neurologic abnormality.
Bed wetting	Considered normal in children until the age of five.
Functional incontinence	Most common in the elderly because of inability to control the bladder related to time and mobility limitations, thinking, and/or communication deficits.
Fecal incontinence	A loss of normal control of the bowel.
Mixed incontinence	More than one type of incontinence; more common in women.
Overflow incontinence	Urination triggered by incomplete emptying of the bladder. A constantly full bladder can lead to weak muscles, causing dribbling.
Stress incontinence	Involuntary leakage related to coughing, laughing, sneezing, or other activities that cause bladder pressure.
Temporary incontinence	Temporary leakage that results from various medical conditions, severe constipation, infections, or medications.
Urge incontinence	A sudden, uncontrollable urge to urinate.

Assist patients with incontinence to obtain medical advice because any type of incontinence can be an indication of a more serious underlying condition. Incontinence can cause patients embarrassment, thereby restricting activities and social interactions and can increase falls and injuries as older patients attempt to rush to the toilet. Incontinence can be caused by many factors such as:

- Stress from exercise, physical activity, coughing, laughing, or sneezing.
- Overactive bladder (OAB)
- Pelvic organ prolapse (POP)

- Pregnancy and childbirth
- Nocturia (frequent urinating during the night)
- Urinary tract infections (UTIs)
- Urinary retention
- Enlarged prostate
- Peyronie's disease
- Irritable bowel syndrome (IBS)
- Inflammatory bowel conditions
- Various neurological conditions such as multiple sclerosis, spinal cord injury, dementia, Parkinson's disease
- Obstruction
- Prostate cancer

Incontinence Products

Numerous products assist with incontinence and give people various options related to their lifestyles and to improve quality of life. In the hospital or skilled nursing facility, various fecal and urinary management systems can be used but require an understanding of indications for use and education regarding proper use of incontinence products.

Incontinence products

- Under pads
- Protective underwear
- Liners
- Pads
- Disposable briefs
- Belted undergarments

Frequent bathing is an easy option that cleanses the body, reduces body odor, provides an opportunity for range of motion, stimulates circulation, and improves self-image. Evidence-based practice still considers bathing the best means for promoting skin integrity.

Fast Facts

Support and educational resources for patients suffering from bowel or bladder incontinence can be found at the National Association for Continence:
http://www.nafc.org

Optimal Skin Care Practices and Prevention Awareness

- Use pillows as a cost-efficient way to support the patient's position and separate and offload bony prominences.
- Enforce a strict 2-hour or less turn and reposition schedule for immobile patients.
- Float the patient's heels off the bed using pillows or other devices such as Prevalon boots.
- Change linens and patient gowns frequently to promote clean, dry skin.
- Moisturize the patient's skin often and apply barrier creams after changing incontinence briefs.
- Prevent shearing and friction on the patient's feet and toes by making a tent with the covers or use a bed cradle.
- Protect the patient's limbs from bedrails by padding the rails.
- Remind a sitting patient to shift position every 15 minutes.
- Use appropriate draw sheets, trapeze, or bariatric-lifting devices when turning and repositioning patients.
- Educate the patient, family, and care providers about:
  - The importance of skin care and prevention of breakdown.
  - Good nutrition maintaining skin integrity and healing.
  - Physical activity and exercise.
- Assess skin daily and intervene immediately if new wounds or breakdown develops.

Bibliography

HPFY. Retrieved from www.healthproductsforyou.com
National Alliance for Continence. Retrieved from https://www.nafc.org

15

Selecting Optimal Support Surfaces and Patient Positioning

INTRODUCTION

In the past, bed frames were strung with ropes. Today, a patient bed is a specialized device known as a support surface, with pressure redistribution being the goal. Choosing the correct support surface to prevent or manage a pressure injury is as critical as the diagnosis. The amount of money spent annually for support surfaces is staggering and so is the complexity of these support surfaces. They range from reactive supports to active supports, integrated bed systems, nonpowered beds, and overlays, to simple standard mattresses. Although the support surface is only one part of a comprehensive treatment plan, it can be crucial to a patient's outcome.

In this chapter, you will learn:

1. National Pressure Injury Advisor Panel (NPIAP) categories, mechanical characteristics, components, and physical concepts of support surfaces.
2. Factors that guide the selection of a support surface.
3. Advantages and disadvantages of support system surfaces.
4. About bariatric equipment.
5. Centers for Medicare & Medicaid Services (CMS) support surface guidelines.

SUPPORT SURFACES

The CMS and NPIAP address support surfaces. Qualifying support surface criteria are essential to choosing the most appropriate surface for the patient and to providing the greatest cost savings to the facility. See Tables 15.1 and 15.2. The NPIAP provides the best evidence-based research available regarding support surfaces, and the CMS guidelines are the most standardized for addressing coverage of support surfaces. The NPIAP and the CMS work together to develop consistent terminology so that standards are uniform.

The CMS classifies support surfaces into three categories:

Group 1

Designed to either replace a standard hospital or home mattress or as an overlay placed on top of a standard hospital or home mattress. Products in this category include:

- Mattresses
- Pressure pads
- Overlays

Table 15.1

NPIAP Categories and Mechanical Characteristics of Support Surfaces	
Support Surface	Definition
Reactive support surface	A powered or nonpowered support surface with the capability to change its load distribution only in response to an applied load.
Active support surface	A powered support surface with the capability to change its load distribution properties with or without an applied load.
Integrated bed system	A bed frame and support surface that are combined into a single unit whereby the surface is unable to function separately.
Nonpowered support surface (static support surface)	Any support surface not requiring or using external sources of energy for operation.
Powered support surface (dynamic support surface)	Any support surface requiring or using external sources of energy to operate.
Overlay	An additional support surface designed to be placed directly on top of an existing surface.
Mattress	A support surface designed to be placed directly on the existing bed frame.

Table 15.2

NPIAP Features of Support Surfaces

Features of Support Surface	Definition
Air fluidizing	A feature of a support surface that provides pressure redistribution by forcing air through a granular medium (e.g., beads) producing a fluid state.
Alternating pressure	A feature of a support surface that provides pressure redistribution via cyclic changes in loading and unloading, as characterized by frequency, duration, amplitude, and rate of change parameters.
Lateral rotation	A feature of a support surface that provides rotation about a longitudinal axis, as characterized by degree of a patient's turn, duration, and frequency.
Low air loss	A feature or a support surface that provides a flow of air to assist in managing the heat and humidity (microclimate) of the skin.
Zone	A segment with a single-pressure redistribution capability.
Multizone	A surface in which different segments can have different pressure redistribution capabilities.

Group 2

Designed to either replace a standard hospital or home mattress or as an overlay placed on top of a standard hospital or home mattress. Products in this category include:

- Powered air flotation beds
- Powered pressure-reducing air mattresses
- Nonpowered advanced pressure-reducing mattresses

Group 3

- Complete bed systems, known as air-fluidized beds, which use the circulation of filtered air through silicone beads.

Fast Facts

The NPIAP defines a support surface as "a specialized device for pressure redistribution designed for management of tissue loads, micro-climate, and/or other therapeutic functions (i.e., any mattresses, integrated bed system, mattress replacement, overlay, or seat cushion, or seat cushion overlay)."

Functional features of a support surface may be used alone or in combination with others.

FACTORS GUIDING SELECTION OF A SUPPORT SURFACE

The Patient

- No person is free from pressure because no person is weightless.
- What does the patient need?
  - More surface area?
  - Contact with the surface to be temporarily removed?
  - Contact shifted to other areas?

Weight and Height of the Patient

- Does the person need a bariatric-sized bed?

Multiple Devices

- Is more than one device needed?
- A morbidly obese patient might need a bariatric bed, lift, and bariatric bedside commode.

Tolerance

- Is the patient comfortable and pain free regarding the support surface?

Independent Functioning

- Some support surfaces interfere with the patient's ability to move off the bed.

Compliance

- Most support surfaces still require that the patient be turned and repositioned.
- Make sure the staff, family, and care providers understand the importance of scheduled repositioning.

Time

- Is the support surface needed for short-term or long-term usage?

Feasibility

- Have the staff, family, and care providers had proper education about the care and proper performance of the equipment?

Equipment Needs

- Is the room large enough to accommodate the equipment? Does it allow care providers to work around the bed?
- Does the room have working electrical outlets? Are their locations convenient for the bed?

Reimbursement

- Is the support surface financially feasible?
- Is there a contract already established with the facility?

RECOMMENDATIONS FOR USE OF SUPPORT SURFACES

The Wound, Ostomy and Continence Nurses Society (WOCNS) task force developed algorithms for use of various support surfaces. See Table 15.3. General recommendations for use of support surfaces are:

1. Persons who meet facility protocol for a low bed frame and who have a pressure injury, or who are at risk for developing a pressure injury, should receive an appropriate support surface.
2. Persons who have medical contraindications for turning should be considered for an appropriate support surface and repositioning with frequent small position shifts.
3. Persons with a new myocutaneous flap on the posterior or lateral trunk or pelvis should be provided with an appropriate support surface. Minimize the number and type of layers between the patient and the support surface.
4. There is no difference between reactive/continuous low-pressure surfaces and active surfaces with an alternating pressure feature regarding efficacy in pressure injury prevention.
5. Persons with Braden mobility subscale scores of 2 or 1 and a Braden moisture subscale score of 4 or 3 should be placed on a reactive/continuous low-pressure support surface or an active support surface with an alternating pressure feature.
6. Persons with Braden mobility subscale scores of 4 or 3, existing pressure injuries on the trunk or pelvis, and two available turning surfaces should be placed on a reactive/continuous low-pressure (air, foam, gel, or viscous fluid) support surface.
7. Persons with Braden mobility subscale scores of 2 or 1 and Braden moisture subscale scores of 4 or 3 should be placed on a reactive/continuous low-pressure support surface or an active support surface with an alternating pressure feature.

Table 15.3

Advantages and Disadvantages of Support System Surfaces		
Surface	Advantages	Disadvantages
Foam	Lightweight, one-time charge, resists puncture, many sizes, low maintenance	Retains heat, not drainage resistant, limited life, fire hazard
Gel-filled	Low maintenance, easy to clean, multiple-patient use, resists puncture	Heavy, expensive
Fluid-filled	Easy to clean, baffle system available	Requires a heater, can leak, can be over or under filled, heavy, transfers are difficult
Air-fluidized	Easy to clean, requires less repositioning, multiple-patient use, low maintenance	Hot, heavy, expensive, noisy, requires frequent monitoring for proper inflation, transfers are difficult
Low air loss	Requires less repositioning, easy to clean, maintains constant inflation, setup is provided by the supplier	Requires a power source, restricts mobility, skilled setup is required, noisy, expensive
Dynamic overlays	Easy to clean, deflate for transfers, reusable pump, multiple-patient use	Assembly required, requires a power source
Mattress replacements	Multiple-patient use, low maintenance, inexpensive options, reduces staff time	Requires a power source, initial expense is high, unknown life of product, may not control moisture adequately

8. Persons with Braden mobility subscale scores of 2 or 1, existing pressure injuries on the trunk or pelvis, and two available turning surfaces should be placed on a reactive/continuous low-pressure support surface or an active support surface with an alternating pressure feature.

9. Persons with Braden mobility subscale scores of 2 or 1, a Braden moisture subscale of 1 with moisture that cannot be managed by other means, along with existing pressure injuries on the trunk or pelvis, should be placed on a reactive/continuous low-pressure support surface with a low air loss or air-fluidized feature.

10. Persons with multiple Stage 2, or large or multiple Stage 3 or 4 pressure injuries on the trunk or pelvis involving more than one

available turning surface should be placed on a reactive support surface with a low air loss or air-fluidized feature.

11. Persons who have Stages 2 to 4 pressure injuries on two or more turning surfaces, or have one or no available turning surfaces, should be placed on an active support surface with an alternating pressure feature or a reactive support surface with a low air loss or air-fluidized feature.

12. Persons with deep-tissue injuries located on the trunk or pelvis should receive strategies that facilitate tissue temperature reduction between the patient and support surface (e.g., turning regimen and a gel surface or alternating pressure/low air loss/ air-fluidized feature).

13. Persons with pressure injuries on the head or upper or lower extremities should be offloaded and may not require a change in the current support surface.

Fast Facts

The term "pressure redistribution" has replaced the prior terminology "pressure reduction" and "pressure relief."

BARIATRIC EQUIPMENT

Long gone are the days when draw sheets, gate belts, and even slide boards were sufficient tools for lifting, transferring, and repositioning patients. To be considered obese, a person must have a body mass index (BMI) of 30 or greater. Obesity continues to trend upward. Statistics based on the 2019 National Health and Nutrition Examination Survey show that 39.6% of adults and 18.5% of children ages 2 to 19 in the United States are obese. Bariatric equipment can prevent injuries related to manually lifting and transferring obese patients. There are many bariatric options to choose from.

Ambulatory Assistance

- Canes
- Crutches
- Walkers
- Rollators
- KCI, Medline, AliMed, Adaptive Specialists

Assessment

- Scales
- Medline, AliMed

Bathing

- Shower chairs and benches
- KCI, Medline, AliMed, Adaptive Specialists

Beds

- There are a variety and ranges, such as cardiac chair position beds, overlay mattresses, and low-air-loss beds that accommodate up to 54 inches width and 1,000 pounds
  - Hill-Rom, KCI, Medline, Adaptive Specialists, Span-America Medical
- Powered beds
  - There are varieties and ranges that can bear up to 700 pounds. They can also have additional features:
    - Air-fluidized
    - Low air loss
    - Pulmonary
    - Silver technology
    - Removable head and foot boards
    - Turn-assist
    - Hill-Rom, KCI, Medline
- Mattresses
  - Powered and nonpowered
  - Overlays
  - EHOB, Encompass, KCI, Hill-Rom, Medline, Southwest, Talley Group

Furniture

- Overbed tables
- Reclining chairs
- Lift chairs
- Medline, Adaptive Specialists, AliMed, EHOB, Encompass, KCI, Span-America, Talley Group

Incontinence

- Briefs
- Bedside commodes
- KCI, Medline, AvaCare Medical, CSA Medical, NorthShore Care

Pressure Redistribution and Support

- Platforms
- Boots
- Heel and elbow protectors
- Wedges

- Rolls
- Briggs, EHOB, Medline, Southwest, Talley Group

    Transporting

- Lifts
- Stretchers
- Transfer benches
- Wheelchairs
- Encompass, Hill-Rom, KCI, Medline, Adaptive Specialists

Fast Facts

Bottoming Out

Bottoming out is the finding that an outstretched hand, placed palm up between the undersurface of the mattress and the patient's bony prominence (coccyx or trochanter), can readily palpate the bony prominence. Test bottoming out with the patient supine, head flat, and again supine with the head slightly elevated and side-lying.

MEDICARE GUIDELINES AND REIMBURSEMENT FOR SUPPORT SURFACES

For any pressure-reducing support surface to be covered by Medicare (and most insurance providers), the following guidelines must be met (and documented):

Group 1

Mattress or Overlay

1. The person must be completely immobile; that is, the patient cannot independently make changes in body position without assistance, or
2. The person has limited mobility; that is, the patient cannot independently make changes in body position significant enough to alleviate pressure and at least one of the conditions as follows, or
3. The person has any Stage 2 pressure injury on the trunk or pelvis and at least one of the following conditions:
   - Impaired nutritional status
   - Fecal or urinary incontinence
   - Altered sensory perception
   - Compromised circulatory status

Group 2

Certain specialty beds, powered pressure-reducing mattresses, non-powered advanced pressure-reducing mattresses

1. The person has multiple Stage 2 pressure injuries on the trunk or pelvis that have failed to improve over the past month, during which time the person has been on a comprehensive treatment program including each of the following:
   - Use of an appropriate group 1 support surface, and
   - Regular assessment by a licensed healthcare practitioner, and
   - Appropriate turning and repositioning, and
   - Appropriate wound care, and
   - Appropriate management of moisture/incontinence, and
   - Nutritional assessment and intervention
2. The person has large or multiple Stage 3 or 4 pressure injuries on the trunk or pelvis.
3. The person has had a myocutaneous flap or skin graft for a pressure injury on the trunk or pelvis within the past 60 days and has been on a group 2 or 3 support surface immediately prior to discharge from a hospital or nursing facility within the last 30 days.

Group 3

Air-Fluidized Beds, Complete Bed Systems

Coverage is limited to bed-ridden or chair-bound patients with Stage 3 or 4 pressure injuries that, without the use of an air-fluidized bed, would be institutionalized.

Bibliography

McNichol, L., Watts, C., Mackey, D., Beitz, J. M., & Gray, M. (2015). Identifying the right surface for the right patient at the right time: Generation and content validation of an algorithm for support surface selection. *Journal of Wound, Ostomy, and Continence Nursing, 42*(1), 5–6. http://dx.doi.org/10.1097/WON.0000000000000103

National Health and Nutrition Examination Survey. (2019). Retrieved from https://www.cms.gov/nchs/nhanes/index.html

Swezey, L. (May 31, 2012). Classes of Support Surfaces. WoundSource, p1. Retrieved from https://www.woundsource.com

United Healthcare Pressure Reducing Support Surfaces Policy Guideline. (2020, May). Retrieved https://www.uhcprovider.com/content/dam/provider/docs/public/policies/medadv-guidelines/p/pressure-reducing-support-surfaces.pdf

IV

Legal Aspects and Regulations

16

Qualifications and Certifications for Wound Care

INTRODUCTION

So, you want to specialize in wound care? The work is hard, and you will encounter many patients undergoing pain and countless hardships because of a chronic or complex wound. Most practitioners either love wound care or they absolutely hate it. I happen to love it, and for those who are intrigued and fascinated with pursuing this labor of love, I have some tips. Wound care requires knowledge of the process of wounds, as well as appropriate judgment in the care and treatment of wounds. The field of wound care management offers a variety of choices, such as hospital-based wound care, hyperbaric medicine, wound ostomy management, outpatient wound clinic care, and consulting. Wound care is a specialty that is diverse and shared by nurses, nurse practitioners, physician assistants, physical therapists, and physicians. Certification is essential, and there are different levels of specialization. The certification process is as individual and unique as the person pursuing the career.

In this chapter, you will learn:

1. The top governing bodies in wound care and what kind of certifications these organizations offer, as well as the requirements for each program.
2. About wound care organizations and associations.

WOUND CERTIFICATION PROGRAMS

Wound care specialization is exciting and rewarding when it is balanced with one's personal goals and career path. Certification demonstrates that you, as a clinician, have specialized knowledge in wound management and that your wound center can provide comprehensive, quality wound care that other healthcare facilities cannot. Wound certification also provides a steppingstone for career advancement. Various certification programs are available for wound care specialization and are described as follows.

Note: Check the organizations' websites for current fees.

The Wound, Ostomy, and Continence Nursing Certification Board (WOCNCB)

- *Eligibility requirements*
  - Registered nurses with a BSN degree (or higher) with a current license
  - Completion of ONE of the following pathways of education or practice:
    - Graduate from an accredited wound, ostomy, and continence (WOC) nursing program within 5 years of seeking certification; programs are listed at: https://www.wocn.org/become-a-woc-nurse/accredited-programs/
    - For each specialty certification sought, 50 CE/CME credits must be completed over the 5 years before applying for certification
    - If you are applying for WOC, a total of 150 CE/CME credits are needed
    - For each specialty certification sought, 1,500 direct patient clinical hours must be completed within the previous 5 years
    - If you are applying for WOC, a total of 4,500 patient clinical hours are needed.
- *Certification credentials:*
  - Certified Wound Care Nurse (CWCN)
  - Certified Wound and Ostomy Care Nurse (CWOCN)
  - Certified Ostomy Care Nurse (COCN)
  - Certified Continence Care Nurse (CCCN)
  - Certified Wound Ostomy Nurse (CWON)
  - Certified Foot Care Nurse (CFCN)
- These certifications are accredited by the National Commission for Certifying Agencies, the American Board of Nursing Specialties, and the WOCN

- Certification is valid for 5 years
- Consider the certification for *Advanced Practice Wound, Ostomy or Continence* if you are an advanced practice registered nurse, nurse practitioner, or clinical nurse specialist
- More information is available at WOCNBC's website: www.wocncb.org

American Board of Wound Management (ABWM)

- *Certified Wound Care Associate (CWCA)*
  - LPN/LVH or other certified healthcare assistant (CAN, CMA)
  - Three years of wound care experience
- *Certified Wound Specialist (CWS)*
  - Licensed healthcare professional with a bachelor's, master's, or doctoral degree
  - Three or more years of wound care experience
- *Certified Wound Specialist Physician (CWSP)*
  - MDs, DOs, DPMs
  - Three or more years of wound care experience
- Annual renewal requires six CE/CME credits
- Certification is valid for 10 years
- More information is available at ABWM's website: www.abwmcertified.org

American Board of Wound Healing (ABWH)

- *Certified Hyperbaric Specialist (CHS)*
  - Minimum of 500 hours of clinical hyperbaric experience per year for the prior 2 years
  - Positions eligible to apply:
    - Hyperbaric technicians
    - Diver medical technician
    - Medical assistant
    - Respiratory therapist
    - Certified nurse aide
    - EMT/paramedic
    - Physician assistant
    - RN/LPN
    - Nurse practitioner
    - Physician
    - Veterinarian
    - Podiatrist
  - Certification is valid for 5 years

- *Physician Certification for Hyperbaric Medicine (FACHM)*
  - Have attained primary board certification in an ABMS-approved specialty and have an active license
  - Minimum of 300 supervised clinical hours in hyperbaric patient treatments
  - Certification is valid for 10 years
  - Annual renewal requires a minimum of 100 hyperbaric patient treatments during the prior 12 months
- *Certified Hyperbaric and Wound Specialist (CHWS)*
  - Minimum of 2 years' experience as a hyperbaric technician with cross-training as wound care assistant or equivalent position
  - Persons eligible to apply are the same as CHS
  - Certification is valid for 5 years
- *Certified Skin and Wound Specialist (CSWS)*
  - Minimum of 2 years' experience as a wound care assistant or equivalent position
  - Minimum of 200 hours of clinical wound training and active experience per year for the prior 2 years
  - Completion of core competencies in wound care
  - Completion of 12 CME/CE credits in wound care
  - Persons eligible to apply are the same as CHS/CHWS
  - Certification is valid for 5 years
- *Physician Certification in Wound Care (FAPWCA)*
  - Eligibility requires MD, DO, DPM with an active license and membership in a professional wound care society
  - Completion of at least 20 CME credits in wound care
  - Recertification requires continued active practice in the field of wound care and is valid for 10 years
  - More information is available at ABWH's website: www.abwh.net

National Alliance of Wound Care and Ostomy (NAWCO)

- *Wound Care Certification (WCC)*
  - Persons eligible to apply
    - RN
    - LPN/LVN
    - Nurse practitioner
    - Physician assistant
    - Physical therapist/occupational therapist
    - PTA/OTA
    - MD/DO/DPM
  - Must meet ONE education requirement
    - Graduation from a skin and wound management education course, **or**

- Current active CWCN, CWON, CWOCN from the WOCNCB, **or**
- CWS from the ABWM, **and**
  - Must meet ONE experience requirement
    - Completed 120 hours of hands-on clinical training in wound care, **or**
    - Completed 2 years' full time or 4 years' part time in wound care
  - Certification is valid for 5 years
- *Advanced Wound Care Certified (AWCC)*
  - Persons eligible to apply are the same as WCC
  - Current active certification as a WCC, WOCNCB, CWCN, CWON, CWOCN
  - Must meet ONE education requirement
    - Completion of an advanced wound training course, **and**
  - Must meet ONE experience requirement
    - One-year full-time or two-year part-time experience with patient care in wound management
  - Certification is valid for 5 years
- *Diabetic Wound Certified (DWC)*
  - Persons eligible to apply are same as AWCC
  - Two-year full-time or 4-year part-time direct patient care with diabetic patients in the past 5 years
  - Must meet ONE pathway requirement
    - Have a published work related to the care of diabetic patients, **or**
    - Serve on a nationally known diabetic organization, **or**
    - Have presented a diabetic topic at a national conference
  - 60 CE/CEU credits in diabetic/wound/nutrition within the last 5 years
  - Completed a diabetic skin and wound management education course
  - Certification is valid for 5 years
- *Nutrition Wound Care Certified (NWCC)*
  - Persons eligible to apply
    - Registered dietician
    - Registered dietician nutritionist
  - One-year full-time or 2-year part-time experience as a dietician
  - Must meet ONE pathway requirement
    - Have a published work related to nutrition in wound care, **or**
    - Serve on a nationally known wound care organization, **or**
    - Have presented a diabetic or wound-related topic at a national conference

- 25 CE/CEU credits in skin and wound care within the last 5 years
- Certification is valid for 5 years
- *Ostomy Management Specialist (OMS)*
  - Persons eligible to apply are the same as AWCC
  - One-year full-time experience in the care of ostomy patients in the last 5 years
  - Must meet ONE pathway requirement
    - Have a published work related to ostomy care, **or**
    - Serve on a nationally known ostomy organization, **or**
    - Have presented an ostomy-related topic at a national conference
  - 60 CE/CEU credits in ostomy and wound care within the last 5 years
  - Completion from a certified ostomy course
  - Certification is valid for 5 years
- *Lymphedema Lower Extremity (LLE)*
  - Persons eligible to apply are the same as AWCC
  - One-year full-time experience in the field within the last 5 years
  - Completion from a certified lymphedema course and 30 CE/CEU credits **or**
  - Active certification as a certified lymphedema therapist and 22 CE/CEU credits
  - Certification is valid for 5 years
- More information is available NAWCO's website: www.nawccb.org

Council for Medical Education and Training

- Persons eligible to apply
  - MD/DO/DPM/DDS
  - Minimum 2 years' experience in wound care
  - Certification is valid for 7 years
  - 24 CME credits specific to wound care required every 3 years
  - More information is available at the Council's website: www.councilmet.org

American Board of Multiple Specialties in Podiatry

- Persons eligible to apply
  - Board-certified podiatrist
  - Certification is valid for 4 years
  - 80 CME credits specific to wound care required every 4 years
  - More information is available at the Board's website: www.abmsp.org

Fast Facts

The Wound Care Education Institute provides industry-leading training both online and in the classroom, as well as annual conferences for CE/CME.

www.wcei.net

Bibliography

ABMSP. Retrieved from https://www.abmsp.org/

American Board of Wound Healing. Retrieved from https://abwh.net/get-certified/

American Board of Wound Management. Retrieved from https://abwmcertified.org

Councilmet. Retrieved from https://councilmet.org/

National Alliance of Wound Care of Ostomy. Retrieved from https://www.nawccb.org/

Wound, Ostomy, and Continence Certification. Retrieved from https://www.wocncb.org/certification/wound-ostomy-continence

17

Facility Accreditation

INTRODUCTION

"Mirror, mirror, on the wall, who's the fairest of them all?" When it comes to a facility's reputation, quality patient care is certainly not subjective. Quality patient care is measured by objective data, which is available to the public. Measured quality care is different than the subjective reputation of a facility.

In your facility, you are one of the creative frontline workers in the trenches, taking responsibility for and administering patient care. You probably also take the rankings of the facility very seriously, often, for instance, playing a role in pressure injury prevention. These empirical rankings are the mirror on the wall. Does this imply that a wound care specialist would not seek a position at a facility with low rankings? Absolutely not! A wound care specialist is passionately driven by excellence, not only providing quality care, but also striving to improve the standard of quality itself. This chapter is dedicated to helping healthcare providers understand who provides the certification and accreditation to healthcare facilities and organizations. A passionate, responsible wound care specialist wants to work in an environment where he or she is driven to excel in the highest standards of safe and effective care.

In this chapter, you will learn:

1. About the Joint Commission and the role with accrediting healthcare facilities.

2. About the American Nurses' Credentialing Center and the magnet program.
3. The other organizations that play a role in the standardization of medical facilities outside the hospital setting.

THE JOINT COMMISSION (JC)

The Joint Commission is a not-for-profit organization that is responsible for hospital accreditation in the United States. Its certification is recognized by most state governments as a requirement of licensure. From 1951 to 2008, the JC was considered the essential body for accreditation, and its accreditation was also recognized as a requirement for healthcare facilities to receive Medicare and Medicaid reimbursement. Since July 15, 2010, the JC's accreditation program has been under the direct authority of the Centers for Medicare and Medicaid (CMS).

Joint Commission FAQs

- All healthcare facilities are subject to a 3-year accreditation cycle (2 years for labs).
- Survey findings are not made public; however, the facility's accreditation decision is.
- Surveys are unannounced.
- Surveyors examine current processes, policies, standards, and procedures, and they must follow JC standards.
- The facility is responsible for updating its standards and expanding patient safety goals on a yearly basis.
- National Patient Safety Goals (NPSGs) provide some of the critical guidelines used to promote and enforce major changes in patient care.

Fast Facts

In 2007, the Joint Commission on Accreditation of Healthcare Organizations (JCAHO) simplified its name to the Joint Commission (JC) and added a logo "Helping Healthcare Organizations Help Patients."

THE AMERICAN NURSES CREDENTIALING CENTER (ANCC)

The American Nurses Credentialing Center is the world's largest and most prestigious nurse credentialing organization, and it is a subsidiary of the American Nurses Association (ANA). The ANCC developed the Magnet Recognition Program to recognize healthcare facilities that provide nursing excellence. Established in 1983 with 41 "magnet hospitals", the ANA developed the Forces of Magnetism, which are characteristics that distinguish magnet hospitals from other hospitals. The vision for magnet hospitals is that they serve as the source of "knowledge and expertise for the delivery of nursing care globally." These facilities are leaders in the reformation of healthcare while sharing a common foundation of magnet principles. To learn more about the ANCC Magnet Program, including a list of magnet hospitals, go to http://www.nursingworld.org.

Outside the Hospital Arena

All external medical facility accreditation programs vary related to cost, clinical standards, skill, and ethical principles. Note, accreditation methods are not the same as government-controlled initiatives. The provision and improvement of healthcare is constantly changing. Whatever accreditation processes that a facility chooses, government-controlled initiatives oversee them. Not all medical facilities use JC accreditation. See Table 17.1.

AMERICAN MEDICAL DIRECTORS ASSOCIATION (AMDA)

The AMDA is an association made up of members from the American Medical Association (AMA) and the American Society of Internal

Table 17.1

National Accreditation Organizations	
Organization	**Description**
Community Health Accreditation Program (CHAP)	assesses community health organizations
Accreditation Commission for Health Care (ACHC)	assesses home health and hospice providers
The Compliance Team	conducts Exemplary Provider Accreditation Programs for durable medical equipment (DME)
Healthcare Quality Association on Accreditation (HQAA)	provides accreditation for home medical equipment providers.
DNV Healthcare	approved by the CMS to accredit hospitals and is sometimes used as an alternative to the JC.

Medicine. The mission of AMDA is to "provide education, advocacy, information, and professional development to promote the delivery of quality long term care medicine." The organization is dedicated to excellence of care for long-term care (LTC) facilities.

AMDA's Overall Goals

1. To be the premier source of information on patient care for LTC facilities.
2. To encourage greater physician involvement in LTC facilities and to develop initiatives.
3. To increase the knowledge base, clinical, skills, and clinical excellence for LTC facilities.

For more information regarding the AMDA's initiatives go to http://www.paltc.org.

THE OUTCOME AND ASSESSMENT INFORMATION SET (OASIS)

For home health agencies to receive payment for Medicare, they must submit a detailed OASIS assessment report on every patient at the following time points:

- Start of care
- Resumption of care following inpatient facility stay
- Recertification within the last five days of each 60-day recertification period
- Other follow up during the home health episode of care
- Transfer to an inpatient facility
- Death at home
- Discharge from an agency

Home health nurses must comply with OASIS standards. The majority of agency patient care (in the home health setting) is 100% covered by Medicare. CMS oversees OASIS regulations. Not adhering strictly to these regulations is detrimental to the financial viability of any agency.

Patients requirements to qualify for Medicare paid home care:

1. The patient must have a physician's order for home care.
2. The patient must be homebound.
3. The patient must need skilled care.
4. The care must be intermittent, temporary, and with a realistic end point.
5. The care required must be reasonable and necessary.

The current version of OASIS (as of January 2019) is called OASIS-D and includes measures of quality of care across post-acute care settings. For more information regarding OASIS-D, go to https://www.cms .gov/Medicare/Quality-Initiatives-Patient-Assessment-Instruments/ HomeHealthQualityInits/OASIS-Data-Sets.

Understanding the Accreditation and Certification Process

It is important for providers seeking employment in a hospital or other facility to do some research and find out who accredits the facility. Knowing this information will make his or her resume stand out. It will indicate to a potential employer the applicant's willingness to partner with the facility to build a reputation of measurable quality care. Wound care clinicians who understand the accreditation and certification process and are willing to work within them are very valuable to their facility.

Bibliography

ANCC. Retrieved from https://www.nursingworld.org/organizational-pro grams/magnet/

The Joint Commission. Retrieved from https://www.jointcommission.org/ about-us/facts-about-the-joint-commission/joint-commission-faqs/

OASIS Data Sets. Centers for Medicare & Medicaid Services. Retrieved from https://www.cms.gov/Medicare/Quality-Initiatives-Patient-Assessment -Instruments/HomeHealthQualityInits/OASIS-Data-Sets

The Society for Post-Acute and Long-Term Care Medicine. Retrieved from https://paltc.org/

18

The Centers for Medicare and Medicaid Healthcare's Common Procedure Coding System

INTRODUCTION

Wound care providers must understand how reimbursement works. The wound care practitioner is paid either hourly or by salary for providing services, applying wound care products, and implementing wound care technology as needed. The facility is reimbursed for the care provided from The Centers for Medicare and Medicaid (CMS) and other related health insurance programs. For the CMS and other related programs to ensure that the claims are processed in an orderly manner, the Healthcare Common Procedure Coding System (HCPCS) was developed.

In this chapter, you will learn:

1. Some reimbursement requirements and guidelines based on the HCPCS.
2. The HCPCS levels.
3. The importance of making cost-effective decisions regarding wound care.
4. Common wound related CPT and HCPCS codes.

HEALTHCARE COMMON PROCEDURE CODING SYSTEM (HCPCS)

The HCPCS is a set of healthcare procedural codes based on the American Medical Association's Current Procedural Terminology (CPT). Established in 1978, the HCPCS provided a standardized coding system for describing specific services and products provided in the delivery of health care. The use of these HCPCS codes, based on health care documentation, became mandatory when the Health Insurance Portability and Accountability Act of 1996 was implemented.

THE THREE HCPCS LEVELS

Level I

Level I codes are maintained by the American Medical Association (AMA). These are Current Procedural Terminology (CPT-4) codes that identify medical services and procedures furnished by physicians and other health care professionals.

- These codes are identifiable as having five numeric digits.
- Procedure codes must match up with the ICD-10 (diagnosis) codes to get claims paid.

Level II

Level II codes are the HCPCS alphanumeric code sets that include non-physician products, supplies, and procedures not included in CPT. See Table 18.1. These generally include non-physician-based services such as:

- Ambulance services
- Prosthetic devices
- Durable medical equipment
- Drugs and supplies
- Non-physician services not covered by Level I codes

Level III

Level III codes (HCPCS local codes) were developed by state Medicare and Medicaid agencies and private insurers for use in specific programs and jurisdictions. Some payers prefer that medical coders report the Level III code in addition to Level I and Level II codes.

Table 18.1

Level II HCPCS Codes for Wound Care Products

Wound Care Product	HCPCS Code
Absorbent dressing	A6234-A6238
Abdominal binder	L1270
Adhesives	A4364
Adhesive bandages	A6413
Adhesive disc or foam pads	A5126
Adhesive remover	A4455-A4456
Alcohol wipes	A4245
Alginate type dressings	A6196-16199
Betadine	A4246-A4247
Cleanser, wound	A6260
Collagen wound dressing	A6020-A6024
Composite dressing	A6200-A6205
Compression bandage	A4460
Compression burn garment	A6501-A6512
Compression stockings	A6530-A6549
Contact layer	A6206-A6208
Elastic garments	A4466
Filler, wound (not classified)	A6261-A6262
Film, transparent	A6257-A6259
Foam	A6209-A6215
Gauze	A6216-A6230, A6402-A6406
Gauze, impregnated	A6222-A6233, A6266
Gauze, non-impregnated	A6402-A6404, A6216-A6221
Hydrocolloid dressing	A6234-A6241
Hydrogel dressing	A6242-A6248, A6231-A6233
Iodine swabs/wipes	A4247
Moisturizer, skin	A6250
Negative-Pressure Therapy Pump	E2402
Negative-Pressure accessories	A6550
Non-contact wound warming cover	E0231-E0232
Protectant, skin sealant, moisturizer	A6250
Specialty absorptive dressing	A6251-A6256
Sterile water	A4216-A4217, A4714
Hyperbaric Oxygen Therapy	A4575
Transparent film	A6257-A6259
Tubular dressings	A6457

WOUND CARE CPT CODES FOR DEBRIDEMENT

Wound debridement codes include 11042-11047. Documentation guidelines for these codes are:

- Report depth of tissue that is removed (epidermis, dermis, subcutaneous, muscle and/or fascia) and surface area of wound.
- Surface area is billed and reimbursed for the first 20 sq cm or less and each additional 20 sq cm thereof.
- For a single wound, report the depth using the deepest level of tissue removed.
- For multiple wounds of the same depth, add the surface area of the wounds.
- For multiple wounds of different depths, report each separately at the deepest level for each.

UNDERSTANDING REIMBURSEMENT GUIDELINES

The coding process is complex, and assignment of an HCPCS code does not imply approval or a guarantee of claim reimbursement. Common reasons for Medicare claims denial are:

- Nonspecific diagnosis codes
  - Always identify and document the source or type of wound
- The medical record did not justify medical necessity
  - Document the exact primary diagnosis, secondary diagnosis, and comorbidities
  - Document the description and size of wounds
    - Photograph wounds before, during, and at conclusion of treatment
  - Document adequate circulation/oxygenation to support wound healing
    - Duplex studies and vascular consults for lower extremity wounds
  - Document details of treatment and response to treatment
    - Edema control
    - Infection control
    - Wound offloading
    - Debridement
    - Management of concomitant medical conditions
    - Use of appropriate dressings to promote wound healing
  - Inaccurate documentation of level of tissue debrided and procedure notes

Fast Facts

Having a Certified Medical Coder is a great asset for a health care provider or facility to employ. Medical Coders specialize in reviewing clinical documentation and assigning correct CPT, ICD-10, and HCPCS codes.

Making Cost-Effective Decisions Regarding Wound Care

It is necessary for the wound care providers to understand the patient's reimbursement plan to promote compliance with the treatment plan. Healthcare providers who show an interest in supply costs balance their care for the patient and the facility that they work for. A good example is barrier creams, which range from $6.00 per tube to upwards of $175.00 per tube. What level of product is necessary, and can the patient afford it?

Become familiar with these reimbursement guidelines:

- What is the patient setting? Is it acute care, home health care, or a skilled nursing facility?
- Who is the paying for the care? Medicare, an HMO, a private health insurance provider, or Workman's Comp?
- What are the coverage benefits, deductibles, and copayments?
- Is the treatment a medical necessity? Does the patient's diagnosis support the medical necessity?
- Do the dressings, services, and technology support the medical necessity?
- Are the codes correctly verified by Medicare or other sources?
- What are the fees or assigned payment amounts for services?

A wound care specialist must understand his or her facility's reimbursement environment because the provider plays an important role in determining what resources and supplies to use for patient care. The wound care specialist must think critically about strategies and responsibilities regarding how his or her decisions and actions generate costs to the facility. Making cost-effective decisions while working within the contractual constraints of the facility will help healthcare providers maximize patient resources.

Communicate with patients regarding the cost of their care. The information a patient provides will facilitate the development of a realistic treatment plan, shed light on other options, involve the patient in decision making, and increase compliance.

Fast Facts

A complete list of HCPCS wound related codes can be found at:
https://www.cms.gov/medicare-coverage-database

Bibliography

Schaum, K. (2015, March). Medicare payment trends and tips. *Today's Wound Clinic, 9*(2), 5–8. Retrieved from https://www.todayswoundclinic .com/articles/medicare-payment-trends-tips

Webb, L. (2012, September 5). Note similarities and differences between HCPCS, CPT codes. Just Coding News. Retrieved from https://www .hcpro.com/HIM-284009-8160/Note-similarities-and-differences -between-HCPCS-CPT-codes.html

Wound Care/CPT Codes for Debridement. Retrieved from https://codingintel .com/wound-care-cpt-codes-for-debridement/

Index